Spiritual Reiki

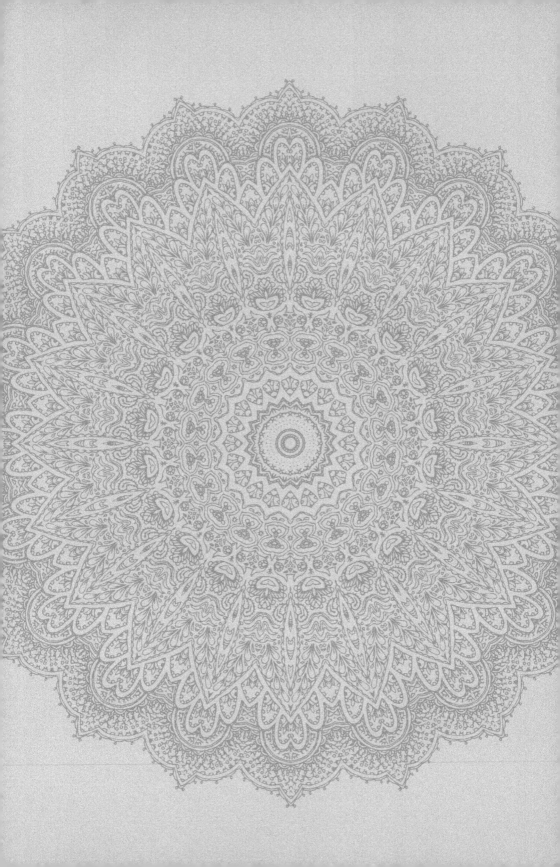

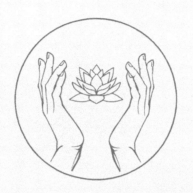

Spiritual Reiki

Channel Your Intuitive Abilities
for Energy Healing

SARAH PARKER THOMAS

Illustrations by Jonathan Bartlett

ROCKRIDGE
PRESS

Interior and Cover Designer: Richard Tapp
Art Producer: Michael Hardgrove
Editor: Clara Song Lee
Production Editor: Ruth Sakata Corley
Illustration © 2020 Jonathan Bartlett
ISBN: Print 978-1-64611-925-7 | eBook 978-1-64611-943-1
R0

This book is dedicated to all the
Reiki healers—past, present, and future.
Together we heal and grow.

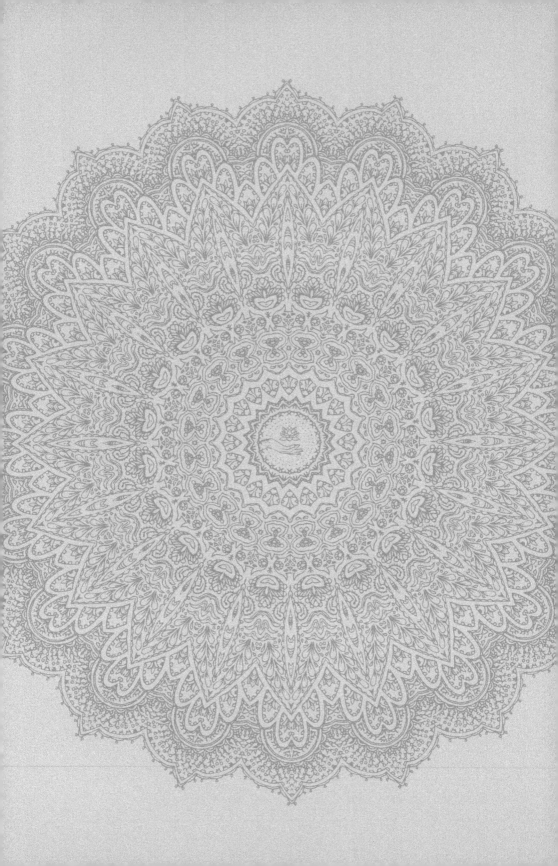

Contents

Introduction ix

PART 1 SPIRITUAL REIKI 1

CHAPTER 1 What Is Reiki? 3

CHAPTER 2 How to Perform Spiritual Reiki 15

CHAPTER 3 Spiritual Reiki 31

CHAPTER 4 Tapping Into Your Spiritual Abilities 47

CHAPTER 5 Enhance Your Spiritual Practice 63

PART 2 TECHNIQUES FOR SPIRITUAL AWAKENINGS AND HEALING 73

CHAPTER 6 Hand Positions for Self-Healing 75

CHAPTER 7 Hand Positions for Healing Others 83

CHAPTER 8 Sequences for Enhancing and Awakening

Spiritual Experiences 101

CHAPTER 9 Sequences for Spiritual and Emotional Healing 125

Resources 162

References 163

Index 164

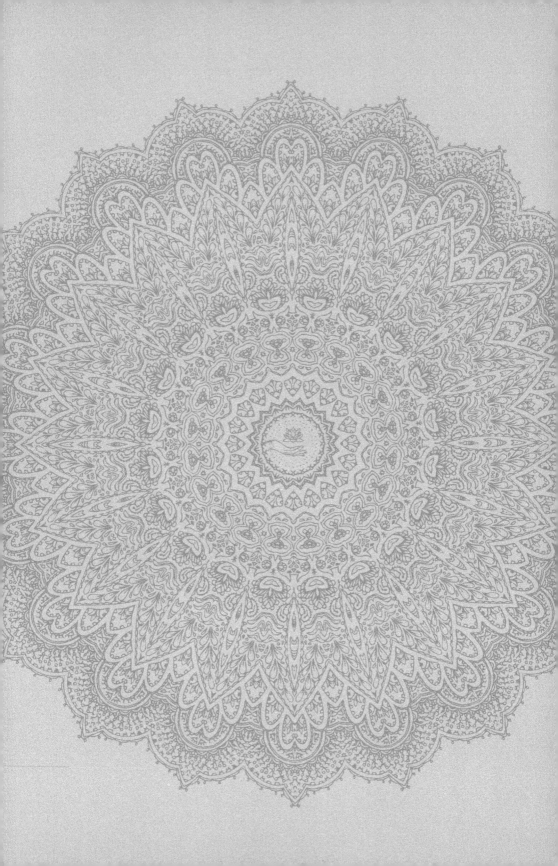

Introduction

Thank you for allowing me to be a part of your spiritual Reiki journey. I am honored and humbled to share this amazing energy with you. I came to Reiki after my husband was suddenly taken from me in a tragic accident. One minute he was here, and then the next he was gone. I was a young mother and the grief was paralyzing. As I struggled with my emotions, it was suggested I take Reiki classes to help me manage the trauma and loss. I was somewhat skeptical Reiki would help, but I was at the end of my rope, so I relented and began my personal Reiki journey.

I should qualify I was born an intuitive and am an empath. My friends thought I was a little bit "witchy" because I collected crystals, practiced yoga, and studied the tarot. I was searching for meaning and a deeper understanding of the synchronicity that flowed all around me, but I could not fully grasp the meaning behind these "random" events.

Little did I know Reiki was the missing piece in my spiritual journey! I never expected the change Reiki would initiate in my life. This phenomenal healing energy is a hands-on modality that is almost impossible to talk about until you experience it. I knew before beginning Reiki classes that everything was made of energy and held a vibration, but after becoming attuned to Reiki, I was able to interact with energy on a completely different level. The very way I viewed energy and events around me changed profoundly. It is normal for Reiki practitioners to have vivid dreams, sense energy, or have sudden flashes of insight. But honestly, I never thought those experiences would happen to me on such a magnified level. Reiki opened my senses to the spiritual world in a whole new way. For example, as an avid gardener, I often visited botanical gardens and plant nurseries, but I never felt life coming from the plants until after my Reiki attunement. I suddenly felt energy coming off the plants in waves and could interact with the organisms in a completely different way.

Reiki also opened the door to the deep personal healing that I knew I needed to address but had spent my entire life running from. This powerful energy helped me become the true me on many levels. Ultimately,

Reiki kept me from being swallowed alive by grief, but the healing didn't stop there.

Reiki also facilitated profound spiritual growth. My ability to manifest had been blocked by grief, and now suddenly I was manifesting and attracting positive experiences into my life. My intuitive powers skyrocketed. With Reiki energy flowing through me, I could easily tap into my own intuition and inner guidance. I intuitively knew what was best for me and what experiences I should let go. Another layer of life was opening up for me, thanks to the magic of Reiki.

This dynamic energy saved me, and I am confident it can support you on your personal healing journey. Reiki helps us come back into balance so that we no longer search outside of ourselves for answers. We learn we have always had the answers and can finally tap into them. This book is intended for people who have been attuned to Reiki. No matter what level or Reiki school you come from, you will be able to take away something valuable from these practices.

With this empowerment, we can harness our own inner guidance with confidence and ease. Reiki heals from the inside out, changing everything. Your experiences with Reiki may differ, but by practicing Reiki and walking this path, you open yourself up to a whole new world of profound and magical experiences. You can expect to feel empowered, grounded, and confident in your day-to-day life.

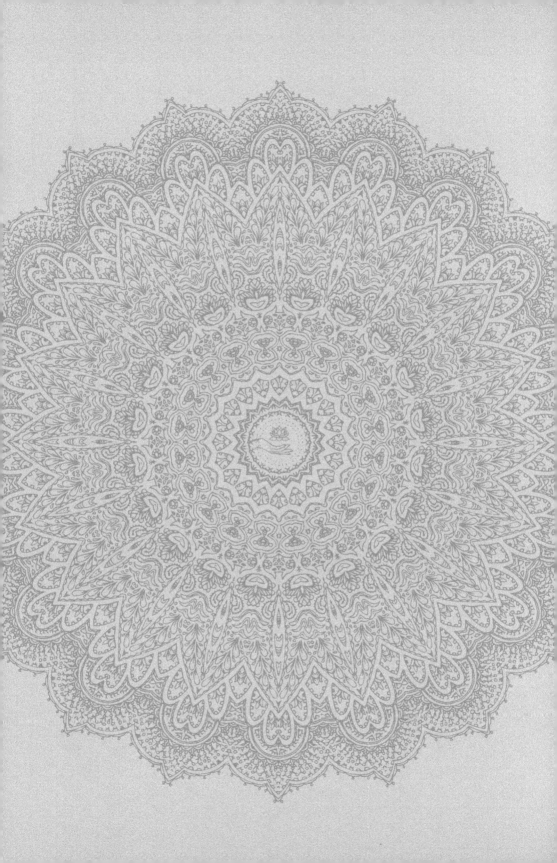

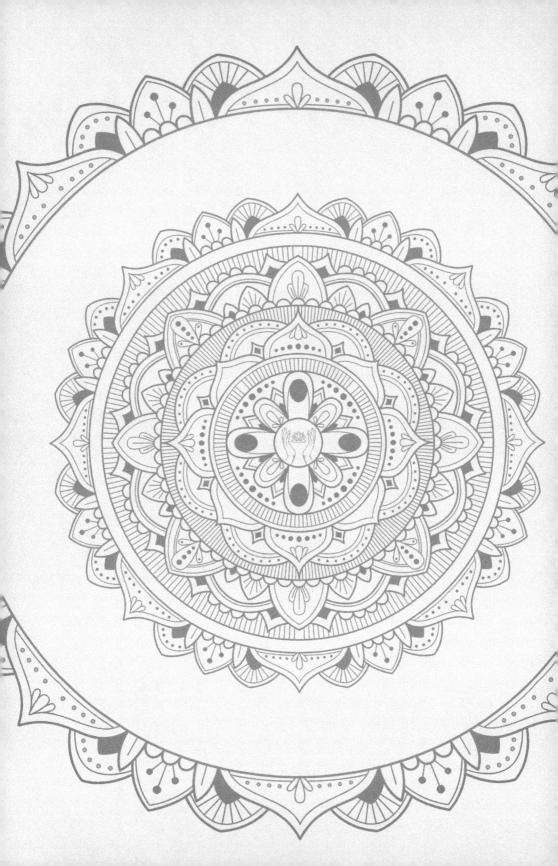

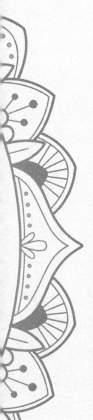

Part 1

Spiritual Reiki

In part 1 of this book, we will explore Reiki and some of the spiritual aspects of this amazing energy. In part 2, we will go over practical steps you can implement to open your Reiki channel. I'll include hand positions, techniques, and empowered exercises to work with. You will learn more about the Reiki symbols and the attunement process, and dive deeper into making Reiki a part of your everyday life.

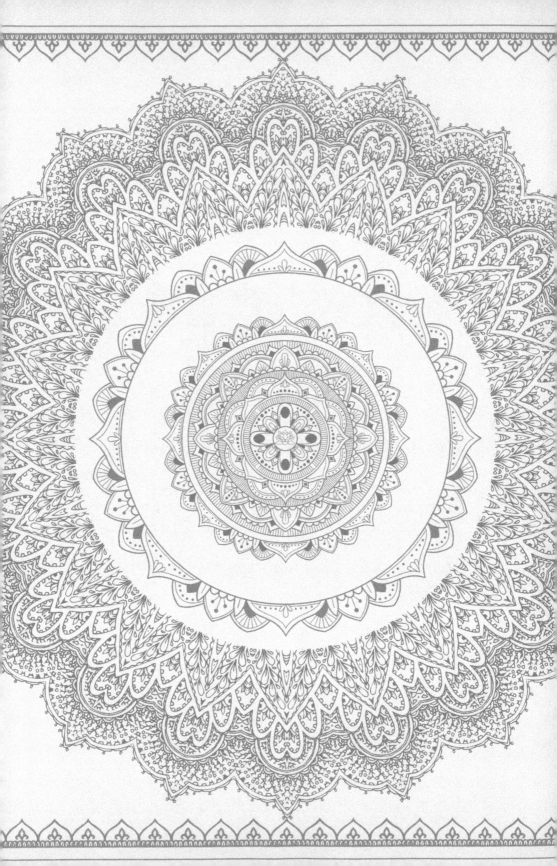

Chapter 1
What Is Reiki?

Welcome to the wonderful world of Reiki. This subtle yet powerful energy isn't a replacement for traditional medicine or a magical cure for disease, but it is a valuable tool in your personal healing arsenal. In this chapter, we will discuss what Reiki energy is, the enigmatic history of Reiki, key historical figures, the evolution of this powerful energy, and the fundamentals of spiritual Reiki. You will learn what to expect in a Reiki class as well as what an attunement consists of and why it is so important. If you are new to the world of Reiki or if you want a quick, concise refresher, begin here.

History

Reiki is a subtle yet dynamic healing energy, quite unlike other types of therapeutic hands-on healing techniques or modalities. Reiki is unique in that it focuses on the personal healing of both the practitioner and the client, and it can be transmitted only via an attunement ceremony.

The attunement ceremony opens the flow of Reiki energy to the student, permanently connecting the student to universal life force energy. We will take a closer look at the attunement ceremony and why it is so important in the following chapter.

Reiki has evolved and adapted since its paradoxical origins in the mid-1800s. While the exact story of its origin is lost, Dr. Mikao Usui (August 15, 1865–March 9, 1926) of Japan is credited with the creation of this healing modality.

Dr. Usui was renowned for his interest in medicine, psychology, and religion. He searched for a healing method open to all, free from religious doctrines or tenets. While studying different types of healing systems, he discovered—or perhaps rediscovered—what would later be known as Reiki.

Dr. Usui would go on to refine working with this vital energy and open a healing clinic in Kyoto, Japan. There, he taught and treated people of all backgrounds. As word spread of his healing success, his practice grew. In 1922, he opened a new clinic in Tokyo. Before Dr. Usui died, he taught several Reiki masters, who, in turn, continued to further the spread of Reiki.

Reiki is not a religion, nor is it filled with tenets or dogma. There is only one set of precepts that we are urged to follow—the Reiki precepts. These elements underscore the belief that practitioners should continue to work on themselves and their spiritual growth.

The precepts, attributed to Dr. Usui, are as follows:

"The secret for inviting happiness through many blessings
The spiritual medicine for all illness
For today only:
- *Do not anger*
- *Do not worry*
- *Be humble*
- *Be honest in your work*
- *Be compassionate to yourself and others*
Do gassho* every morning and evening.
Keep them in your mind and recite them for improvement of mind and body."

These precepts were intended to be performed daily by the practitioner. As we sit in meditation, repeat the precepts, and give thanks for our many blessings, we further our personal healing. This practice mitigates our own trauma, promoting a deep spiritual awaking.

*Gassho translates to "hands pressed together in front of your chest."

KEY FIGURES

Many people played pivotal parts in bringing Reiki forward. Unfortunately, the history of Reiki has been obscured by the method of Reiki's initial transmission. Reiki history was passed down as private, oral history. We do know, though, of a handful of historical figures who kept Reiki alive and growing.

As mentioned earlier, Dr. Usui, also known as Sensei Usui, is recognized as the founder of Reiki. It is believed he trained many students, but only a very few went as far as Shinpiden (master/teacher level). One of his students, Dr. Chujiro Hayashi (September 15, 1880–May 11, 1940), started his own branch of Reiki, Hayashi Reiki Kenkyukai. He further developed Reiki by adding additional hand positions, refining the attunement process, and adopting a more formal training protocol. Dr. Hayashi, in turn, trained more Reiki masters, including Hawayo Takata (December 24, 1900–December 11, 1980), who is credited with bringing Reiki to America. In 1940, Dr. Hayashi performed seppuku, or ritual suicide, rather than take part in the bloodshed of the upcoming war. Being a naval reserve officer, Dr. Hayashi knew he would be called to active duty, so rather than participate in the war, he took his own life. His actions say much about his character and personal ethics. Dr. Hayashi passed leadership of his branch of Reiki to Mrs. Takata, probably so that Reiki would survive, as Mrs. Takata was able to flee Japan and go to America before the war.

Almost all of what we know about Reiki today came from the stories passed on from Mrs. Takata, such as her story of being deathly ill and coming to Dr. Hayashi's Reiki clinic for treatment after traditional medicine had failed her.

We should honor and give thanks to all the Reiki teachers and unsung heroes of Reiki. Each played a part in the history of this amazing healing gift, but we should not get so caught up in the history that we forget the message. Reiki is about wellness, empowerment, and healing. There has been some division in the Reiki community over the history and correct techniques for performing a traditional Reiki session, as well as the best way to move forward while staying true to Sensei Usui's vision.

Reiki has gone through a metamorphosis over the course of the last century. This natural transformation is part of the reason Reiki is still being practiced today.

REIKI TODAY

Reiki continues to grow and evolve even today. You might find Reiki at a private clinic, a public hospital, or a county fair. Reiki has become less mystical and more practical for most practitioners. As more scientific studies are conducted on Reiki and as the evidence grows, more established medical facilities, such as Duke Integrative Medicine and New York–Presbyterian Hospital, have come to offer Reiki as a complementary therapy.

Although the fundamentals Sensei Usui envisioned still guide Reiki, some of the secrecy has been lifted. Reiki is no longer considered mystical or limited to only a select few who could find a teacher. Today, some colleges offer Reiki courses with certification programs. Many private individuals also teach Reiki in person or online as a self-paced study. Depending on the teacher, the personal development and spiritual discipline may be left out of Reiki classes in favor of a more "logical" approach with an emphasis on learning hand positions and symbols. This approach is similar to the stance some yoga centers and modern dojos or martial arts studios have adopted, making the decision to teach the physical aspect of martial arts and limiting or omitting the spiritual aspect. It's always wise to discuss the approach a Reiki teacher takes before you enroll in a class.

As different types of Reiki have developed over time, other components have been added to the traditional curriculum. For instance, one may learn about crystal healing, clearing space, dowsing, or essential oils. There are also new Reiki schools that focus on animal Reiki, ascended master Reiki, and elemental Reiki.

The ranking system, or level of mastery, has also changed as more types and schools of Reiki have emerged. Sensei Usui's students studied for years at his clinic before moving up levels. Now, depending on what school you attend, you could become certified in as little as a weekend. Although I do not recommend these programs, they show how much Reiki has changed.

Reiki Basics

Learning Reiki is one of the most liberating and empowering things you will ever do for yourself.

Reiki is not like any other type of energy healing modality available today. It is very simple to learn, but don't be fooled, the benefits are life changing! Reiki is a hands-on healing modality that does not require actual touch. It focuses on sending energy to the body for optimum health. Reiki also differs from other healing techniques in that it works on both the practitioner and the client.

Reiki can be used for pain management, preventive care, and mental/emotional issues ranging from anxiety to addiction, as well as for a host of other issues. Reiki focuses on healing not only the physical symptoms and discomfort associated with illness but also the root cause.

Reiki requires no belief system. It is free from religious doctrines, and it will work to alleviate most mental, physical, and spiritual issues. Reiki, at its core, assists the body in healing itself.

- Reiki isn't a religion, cult, or brotherhood.
- Reiki can be learned at any stage of life.
- Reiki requires no previous training.
- Reiki does not require belief to work.

Reiki requires only a commitment to learning and practice. You do not need to agree to any other dogma.

Reiki is considered an intelligent energy, which means it does not have to be sent to an ailment or problem area. The Reiki energy will direct itself to the affected area and the root cause of the imbalance.

Another way Reiki differs from other healing modalities is that it charges practitioners to commit to working on their own personal healing. By following the Reiki precepts and practicing daily self-Reiki sessions and meditation, the practitioner becomes more balanced and spiritually open.

Reiki is also unlimited energy. Unlike other finite, energy-healing modalities, such as pranic healing or energy-focused healing, there is no limit to the amount of Reiki that can be channeled for a wellness session. When the recipient has received enough of this subtle energy, the body simply (and autonomously) drops the energetic connection and stops accepting the energy.

An Inherently Spiritual Practice

Reiki, like most things in life, flourishes with proper attention. When you fully commit to Reiki and practice daily, your life changes. As your body returns to a balanced state, your health improves and your personal spiritual abilities grow and multiply.

Reiki works directly on all the chakras, or energy centers of the body, giving each what it needs for optimum health and empowerment. By consistently devoting time and energy to your Reiki practice, you develop an empowered spiritual routine.

When we are in the flow of Reiki, we notice magic all around us. Life seems to flow easier, and we become more receptive to it. Our spiritual abilities become second nature. We smile more and embrace a more compassionate view of the world.

Most Reiki students report realizing new spiritual abilities after the initial attunement ceremony and upon completing each additional level of training. Such abilities could include clairvoyance, clairaudience, or other psychic skills. All spiritual experiences have merit and should never be discounted just because you aren't experiencing what you think is "normal." Your personal awakening happens as it is destined to, in the correct time and order. As you sit in gassho and learn to live by the Reiki precepts, you may experience a deeply profound spiritual awakening, or it may happen later while you are doing a mundane chore. Regardless, Reiki is constantly working to assist you on this journey.

Reiki is an inherently spiritual practice, and while it cannot be rushed, embracing Reiki and making it part of your daily routine will encourage a powerful spiritual transformation.

QI AND ENERGY HEALING

Qi, *chi*, *prana*, and *ki* are all names for energy. *Reiki* translates roughly into two Japanese words: *rei*, which means "universal or higher power," and *ki*, which is "life force energy." *Reiki*, then, means "spiritually guided life force energy."

Scientists and gurus agree that everything and everyone is made up of energy. We are beings of energy, moving through and surrounded by energy. Reiki is unlimited life force energy that can be channeled for healing purposes.

Another way of looking at Reiki energy is to compare it to the breaking or tearing energy used in most martial arts. We have all seen martial artists break concrete blocks with their fists. In that context, energy is used to break the bricks. We can all agree if the force were simply strength, anyone could do it. But we know that what breaks the blocks is as much energy as it is brute force. Reiki is that same energy but used on the other end of the spectrum. Instead of breaking and tearing, Reiki restores, balances, and heals.

Energy healing aims to promote health through the manipulation of energies. Most alternative healing modalities believe that illness begins as disturbances in the energy field. Having been attuned and trained in Reiki, the practitioner uses designated hand positions, along with intuitive abilities, to transmit energy to the client's body. This energy then rebalances and restores the body as it works on the chakras, meridians, and energy pathways of the body. We'll discuss this process more later as we dive deeper into chakras and the part they play in our overall wellness.

Reiki is an intelligent energy that does not need to be directed or micromanaged; we often witness Reiki target areas where it is most needed. It is not uncommon to treat someone's foot, for instance, while the person experiences heat, tingling, or other sensations in the arms or shoulders.

SPIRITUAL REIKI

Spiritual Reiki can be thought of as a byproduct of committed Reiki practice. When we commit to a daily Reiki practice, we commit to personal wellness. The more we work with Reiki, the more healing we receive and the more we evolve. It is an awakening process. Suppressed abilities and gifts awaken as we further our own personal healing. Reiki is itself a spiritual practice.

We will discuss this spiritual aspect more in-depth in later chapters, but know that just by reading this book, you are walking the path of spiritual Reiki.

Although Reiki isn't a replacement for conventional medicine or medical care, it can greatly complement it! Reiki can help you manage pain levels, reduce recovery time, and ease side effects from medical treatments.

WHO CAN PERFORM REIKI

Anyone of any age, nationality, or religion can perform Reiki. You do not need to be born with a "gift." Reiki can be learned by anyone at any point in life. But you do need to have some formal training in the basics in order to perform Reiki. You cannot just pick up a book and do it.

The only prerequisite to performing Reiki is that the student must be attuned to Reiki by a teacher who also has been attuned to this energy. After attunement, the student needs a teacher or at least a support group of other practitioners to learn the basics from. I often encounter people who were gifted a Reiki attunement or went to a Reiki weekend course but have no idea how to proceed. The instructor usually suggests students read up and practice, but I find there is too much information for this advice to be effective. Reiki classes can be taken online or in person. They should cover at least the basics of energy medicine, hand positions, working with symbols, ethics, and accountability.

ATTUNEMENT

The attunement process is essentially locking the Reiki energy into the participant and connecting them via lineage to all of the other Reiki healers—past, present, and future.

During your first Reiki class, you will be given a Reiki attunement. Usually a mini-Reiki session is given to each student during the attunement process. Students sit quietly in a meditative state while the Reiki teacher performs the attunement ceremony. This ritual includes energetically placing the Reiki symbols in their auras, balancing and opening their chakras, and permanently linking the students to the Reiki energy. As you move up Reiki levels, you will receive another symbol and attunement.

Participants often report having a powerful spiritual awakening during the ceremony. Seeing guides, past lives, vivid colors, symbols, and other images during an attunement is common. Sensing the presence of relatives who have passed on or ascended masters (spiritually enlightened beings), and hearing unexplained sounds or smells often occur during the ceremony. It is thought that each student's guide or angel is present for the ritual, and many people report sensing a presence.

DEGREES OF REIKI

Sensei Usui introduced these traditional Reiki levels:

Shoden (Beginner—Level 1)

Okuden (Hidden Teachings—Level 2)

Shinpiden (Master/Teacher—Levels 3 and 4)

Today, there are over 100 types of Reiki being taught. Each system has its own protocols and methodology, including new ranking systems and degrees. Individual schools have their own approach to the curriculum, which can also vary greatly from teacher to teacher.

LEVEL 1
BEGINNER

Your experience will be as unique as you are, but often at level one, the Reiki student attends classes taught by a certified Reiki teacher. Students learn the history of Reiki, hand positions, general information regarding the meridians, the aura, and the seven major chakras, and they are given an energy attunement. This attunement locks the Reiki into the energy field and makes it possible for the student to access Reiki at any time.

Most, but not all, Reiki schools also include one Reiki symbol at this level. (We will discuss the symbols in the next chapter.) Students learn the Reiki precepts, the foundation of the spiritual side of Reiki, and begin a personal healing journey.

At this point, the Reiki is mainly working on restoring and healing the individual. Although it is possible (and you are encouraged) to practice on others, this time is mainly one of personal awakening and inner healing.

At level one, the student also begins a 21-day detox following the attunement process. Reiki now flows nonstop through the body. Students may feel wonderfully alive and more whole than ever. Colors are brighter, food smells and tastes better, and there is new zest for life!

But not everyone has such an intense or positive experience. Some people also report flu-like symptoms as the body/energy field begins the detoxing period. The body begins to purge fears, anxiety, old thought forms, outdated beliefs, conditioning, and built-up toxins. If this is your experience, take it easy, drink more water, and listen to your body.

Another common side effect from the Reiki attunement is dormant spiritual abilities either suddenly awaken or are given a major power-up. It is not uncommon to experience prophetic dreams, sense energy, and generally be more open to the world after the attunement ritual.

Whatever you experience after a Reiki attunement, know that it is what you were meant to undergo for your own distinct growth and evolution.

LEVEL 2
HIDDEN TEACHINGS

At level two, depending on the Reiki school, the practitioner will attend classes (ideally in person) to review the first level and learn about mental/emotional healing, long-distance healing, and sending Reiki energy to the past and future. Students will be given another attunement, additional hand positions, and new symbols. More information on the chakras is given, as well as instructions for breaking addictions. Depending on the Reiki school, some students also learn crystal healing at this level.

Students' spiritual abilities usually skyrocket at this level. They report becoming more intuitive, experiencing a greater sense of internal knowing, and beginning a spiritual ascension process. They feel more connected to nature, have more compassion, and can see the bigger picture behind life challenges. This stage is also when most students suddenly release negative habits, such as gambling, smoking, or alcohol abuse.

LEVEL 3
REIKI MASTER

At the Reiki master level, most schools include another symbol and attunement. Students will review past classes; show they have an accurate, working knowledge of Reiki; and learn new hand positions. They will learn more about the elements, techniques for addressing more intense ailments, traditional Chinese medicine, and additional techniques for directing Reiki.

At this level, the possible connections among hauntings, spirits, ghosts, and personal health will be addressed. Alternative medicine will be discussed as students learn how to incorporate other modalities into Reiki sessions and the pros and cons of doing so.

A major spiritual awakening usually takes place after the attunement at the Reiki master level. Most people, if they haven't already, connect to and work with guides or angels. They also sense energy and see colors and smells on a much deeper level. Precognitive dreams, inner knowing, and the ability to manifest are usually ramped up. Often, the Reiki master has a personal awakening and a deeper understanding of their life's purpose. Students may suddenly find peace with childhood anguish or other trauma. Their spiritual senses blossom, and they often give up destructive or negative habits and addictions with ease. Most report being happier and more at peace than ever before.

LEVEL 4
REIKI TEACHER

Not all Reiki schools have a teacher level. Some incorporate a teacher level into the Reiki master degree, while other schools have a separate course for teachers.

At this level, students should be able to consistently feel energy and easily distinguish chakra imbalances. A Reiki teacher should be able to easily answer common questions on Reiki and teach from personal experience as well as from a syllabus.

At this point, the Reiki masters or teachers will have had several pivotal spiritual awakenings. Their esoteric knowledge and practical experience will be instrumental in assisting others on this journey.

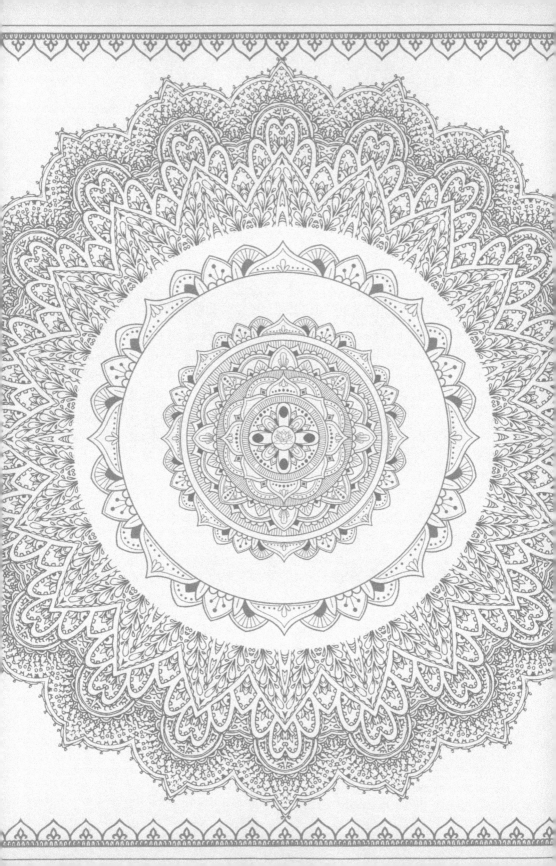

Chapter 2
How to Perform Spiritual Reiki

In this chapter, we will go over the basics of Reiki and its spiritual side. You'll learn how to incorporate Reiki into your everyday personal care routine as you make it the core of your spiritual practice. For almost two decades, I have had the pleasure to witness firsthand how Reiki works in relieving pain, removing debilitating energy blocks, and revitalizing the body. This powerful energy is also instrumental in igniting the flame of spiritual change and awakening dormant abilities.

Energy Healing

Reiki is a safe, gentle, noninvasive form of natural energy healing that is easy to learn. It is considered a complementary, rather than alternative, medicine in most countries.

During a Reiki session, the practitioner channels unlimited life force energy from the Universe to the client. The practitioner delivers the healing energy to the client's body without touch or with light touch. Practitioners may either gently place their hands on the client's body or hold their hands several inches above it. They give special attention to particular locations, such as the seven major chakras or any area that is causing the client pain or distress. There are routine hand positions and techniques for sending energy to combat blockages or underactive energy centers.

The length of time that practitioners leave their hands in each position is determined by the flow of energy, or lack thereof, at specific body locations.

Balancing your energy, removing blocks, and aiding the body in healing itself is the goal of Reiki. Most mind-body practices, such as yoga and tai chi, share the same belief system and are designed to help people achieve internal wholeness and balance. Energy healing is not a new concept, but it does empower the body to return to a state of authentic wellness.

Chakras

Chakra is a Sanskrit word that translates to "wheel" or "disk." It describes a spiritual energy center found within, or above, the human body. We experience the world based on the state of our seven major chakras. These powerful energy centers regulate and dictate our life experiences, including our emotional state, creative abilities, and physical and mental health. The chakras are also key in developing our spiritual abilities.

Each of these major chakras governs a specific part of the physical and emotional body. Each is associated with an element, color, and sound. The seven energy centers also correlate to specific mental and emotional states. We must work to keep the chakras healthy and balanced for optimum health. There are many wonderful books written on the chakra system, containing a trove of information on balancing and aligning these powerful centers. Let's briefly examine how each chakra relates to spiritual Reiki.

ROOT CHAKRA

The *muladhara*, or root chakra, is located at the bottom of the tailbone and is associated with our basic needs, fears, and survival. It is the base of the chakra system and lays the foundation for our physical life. A healthy root chakra is vital to those who are working on their spiritual path.

If the root chakra is blocked or not functioning correctly, the energy necessary for spiritual development will not flow. For the higher chakras to flourish, the root chakra needs to be functioning and healthy.

SACRAL CHAKRA

The *svadhisthana*, or sacral chakra, is located a few inches below the belly button. This energy center is associated with the color orange and governs passion, self-expression, creativity, power, and pleasure. If you are worried about expressing your psychic abilities for fear of being judged, work on balancing this power center. This chakra is also key in learning to trust your intuitive powers.

SOLAR PLEXUS CHAKRA

The *manipura*, or solar plexus chakra, is located in the upper abdomen two inches above the navel. This chakra is associated with the color yellow and is the core of your personality, willpower, and identity. When balanced, this chakra allows you to authentically step into your power and embrace your spiritual abilities.

HEART CHAKRA

The heart chakra, or *anahata*, is associated with the color green and governs our ability to love, show compassion, forgive, grieve, and hope. This chakra is the bridge between the lower, more physically grounded chakras and the higher spiritual energy centers. This energy center is key in opening latent spiritual abilities.

THROAT CHAKRA

The *vishuddha*, or throat chakra, is located at the center of the neck, in the hollow of the throat. It is associated with the color aquamarine and governs our ability to manifest, communicate, and authentically express ourselves. This chakra is also key in connecting with the higher ethereal realms and in empowering our intuitive abilities.

THIRD EYE CHAKRA

The third eye chakra, or *ajna*, is the sixth chakra. It is located in the center of the head and associated with the color indigo. When opened with Reiki and properly balanced, the third eye chakra can allow one to access hidden information, see illness in auras, and access higher consciousness. Clairvoyance, astral projection, mediumship, and other abilities open when this chakra is fully engaged with Reiki.

CROWN CHAKRA

The crown chakra, also known as *sahasrara*, is seen as violet or pure white in color and sits above the crown of the head. By empowering this chakra, we can fully access inner wisdom, understanding our connection to the planet and all life forms. Using Reiki to heal and balance this chakra will open up new spiritual experiences and feelings of bliss and enlightenment.

ADDITIONAL CHAKRAS

In addition to the seven major chakras, there are some other, lesser-known chakras that are very helpful to know for Reiki work.

HARA CHAKRA

The hara is not a chakra in the strict sense of the word but so much more. It is located on the navel or about two finger widths below it but is visualized as an internal spot. This powerful energy spot is more a gateway than a chakra; in Reiki and the healing arts, we know it is a limitless spring of energy. The hara is your center of gravity and your strength to rise above material concerns. Nurturing this chakra is essential for spiritual development.

CHAKRAS IN THE HANDS AND FEET

Two of the most important chakras are located on the palms of the hands and the bottoms of the feet. Your hands have multiple chakras, but the primary chakra is in the center of each palm. This chakra will continue to grow the more you practice Reiki and is integral to sensing and understanding energy. Symptoms of a blocked hand chakra include arthritis, carpal tunnel syndrome, writer's block, an inability to create, an inability to sense energy, and an inability to feel crystals.

Symptoms of a closed foot chakra include insomnia, fatigue, anxiety, restlessness, and mental fog. Opening this chakra can also speed up the body's healing abilities and recovery time, and help people regain their zest for life. Every full Reiki session should include working on the hands and feet for optimum health and wellness.

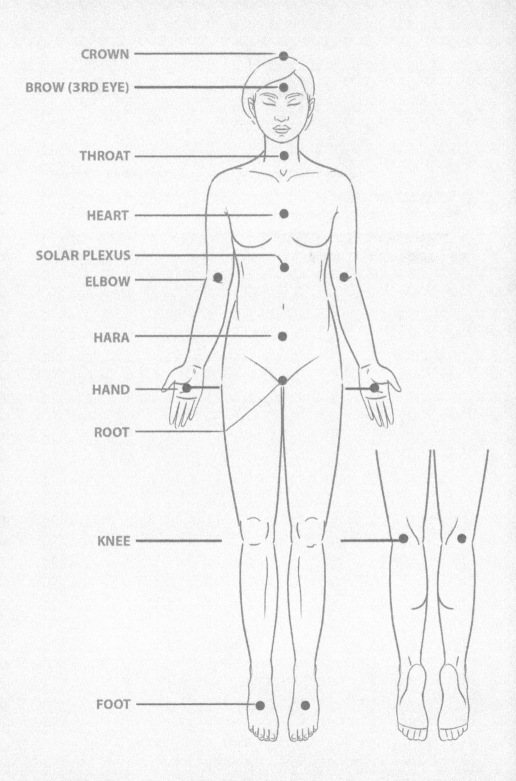

CROWN

BROW (3RD EYE)

THROAT

HEART

SOLAR PLEXUS

ELBOW

HARA

HAND

ROOT

KNEE

FOOT

Hand Positions and Sequences

Hand positions are a large component of modern Reiki. Most healing sessions include distinct sequences for specific ailments, supporting the chakras, and easing physical or emotional pain.

Although it is important to learn proper hand positions, over time we learn to stop overthinking sessions and hand sequences, and just go with the flow. Don't hesitate to practice Reiki because you are unsure if you are doing the hand positions correctly. Reiki is intelligent energy that can do no harm. It will travel to the affected area of the body, even if your positions are slightly off. You cannot harm anyone by placing your hand in a wrong position.

I have included a few hand positions later in the book to give you an idea of where to begin, but as your practice of Reiki grows, you could be led to modify or incorporate your own hand positions.

HANDS-ON HEALING

In a Reiki session, the practitioner delivers energy to the client via light touch or by hovering their hands a few inches above the client's body. (Reiki is done fully clothed, unlike massage.) During the healing session, no massage or physical manipulation is needed; the subtle energy flows to the affected areas of the body of its own accord.

Remember, Reiki is an intelligent energy that will direct itself to the affected area and the root cause of the imbalance. The client's body will pull the energy directly from the practitioner's hands and direct the flow of energy.

DISTANCE HEALING

Being able to send Reiki healing energy long distance is one of the many wonders of Reiki. There are many different methods of doing this; it usually comes down to the Reiki master's preference.

Here are some of the easiest techniques:

- **Use an empowered Reiki box.** You build Reiki boxes by infusing simple boxes with Reiki, applying the symbols, and placing the names of people who have given permission to receive Reiki inside. You can then place the box in a crystal grid or send Reiki to the box.
- **Send Reiki via a photograph.** Many people use this method for sending long-distance healing. Take a photograph of the person who wants to receive long-distance Reiki and write the person's name, age, location, and medical/emotional problem on the back. You then can send Reiki to the picture using the power and the long-distance symbols.
- **Use a surrogate or stand-in for the client.** The power and long-distance symbols are both used in this method. Select a surrogate (such as a stuffed animal) and send Reiki to it while keeping a clear vision of the intended recipient in your mind.
- **Create a Reiki grid.** For this method, you build a crystal grid with Reiki-infused stones to send energy continuously to a recipient.

You can also hold an image of the person in your mind and beam Reiki to the recipient using the long-distance symbol.

We never perform distance healing without prior consent. Some have said that we should just send Reiki and the intended recipient's higher self will either allow it or refuse it. This practice is irresponsible and lazy. If we cannot make the time to ask people if they want the healing, then we should not presume to know what's right for them and send Reiki. Not everyone will want Reiki and that's okay—people have a right to spiritual autonomy, and we should not judge their decisions. Healing takes time and space. We should never force Reiki on anyone.

Who Can Receive Reiki?

Reiki is safe for infants, children, animals, and just about everyone!

Reiki can be very helpful for people who are recovering from illness, surgery, or emotional pain. (Remember, Reiki doesn't replace traditional medical care but complements it.)

As mentioned earlier, we should always ask for permission before sharing Reiki. The general rule is we treat those who cannot ask for or refuse Reiki in person (not long distance) and give them the opportunity to pull away or walk away when they are done receiving the energy. We never force Reiki or healing on anyone. Make sure all your clients can walk or pull away if they do not want to receive the energy. If you are treating infants, young children, people with impairments, or animals, assure that they have consented, or if they're not able to give consent, give them the opportunity to move away. If they have not pulled away from the energy, allow them to decide when the session is over. For example, animals and small children may walk away once they've had their fill, and infants may get fussy or cry when they are done. Once they have moved away or shown signs they have had enough, end the session, even if it has only been a few minutes.

You may notice that children and animals will flock to you now that you are a Reiki person. Dogs and cats may sit under your chair or on your lap, and larger animals may pay much more attention to you. Animals love Reiki!

When treating those who can't ask or decline, such as animals or small children, we always begin the treatment in a relaxed, open area. We allow children and animals space to walk or pull away when they have had enough, which is why we don't treat animals in cages.

Symbols

The Reiki symbols are an intricate part of traditional Reiki. The symbols we use today in traditional Usui Reiki were developed by Sensei Usui. It is believed that Mrs. Takata taught that the Reiki symbols were not to be shown openly to anyone not attuned to Reiki, and most Reiki clinics do not openly display the symbols. However, it is now possible to find the symbols online, in books, and even on merchandise.

The four symbols used in traditional Reiki are the power symbol, the mental/emotional symbol, the long-distance symbol, and the master symbol. The symbols are not Japanese kanji and do not translate into proper words. Each symbol is important in Reiki and allows the practitioner to focus the energy in very specific terms. For example, the power symbol is used to focus the energy on a certain area of the body or on an object. The mental/emotional symbol is used to address emotional issues rather than physical ailments, and the long-distance symbol is used to send Reiki long distance. (Time and space are no longer barriers for healing when using this symbol.) The master symbol enacts a change in the mind of the master as it accesses a different aspect of this powerful energy and allows the master to function at a higher level of consciousness.

When referring to the Reiki symbols by name, we usually refer to the kotodama (the Japanese belief that mystical powers dwell in words and names). When we refer to or discuss the symbols, we use their English names, such as "power symbol" or "long-distance symbol" rather than the actual name of the symbol. The actual names of the symbols are considered sacred sounds empowered with energy.

> **The Power Symbol—Cho Ku Rei:** This is the first symbol learned and the most widely used. We use this symbol to increase power and focus Reiki on a specific spot.
>
> **The Mental/Emotional Symbol—Sei He Ki:** This symbol is used for mental and emotional healing, taking away bad habits, and improving relationships. This powerful symbol can also initiate a healing crisis, and it brings up what needs to be healed.

The Long-Distance Symbol—Hon Sha Ze Sho Nen: This symbol is used to cross time and space. We use it to send energy long distance and backward or forward in time.

The Master Symbol—Dai Ko Myo: This symbol, used only by a master or teacher, is used in attunements, to increase the power of the other symbols, and to assist in connecting one to the higher self.

The purpose of keeping the symbols hidden is so that when a practitioner uses the symbols, only the divine meaning is linked to the image. When symbols of any kind are shown over and over, they become ingrained in our minds and may have many different meanings, depending on how they are used. For instance, the smiley face symbol is now linked to Walmart, but what did you think of when you read the words *smiley face*? The smiley face has been linked to movie characters, happiness, and more in the past. (It actually dates back to an insurance company in Massachusetts.) It is important when we invoke the Reiki symbols that the intended meaning be clear in our minds and free from other associations.

USING SYMBOLS

Each of the Reiki symbols has its own divine use, and as you are attuned to each, you will learn its meaning and purpose. There are many ways to work with the Reiki symbols. Often, they are drawn in the air or envisioned over parts of the body during a Reiki treatment. They can also be printed on affirmations, blown through the air, or written on the bottom of your Reiki table if you so have one.

Once you are attuned to Reiki, you will learn how to draw the symbols at each degree. When you have mastered the symbols, you can use them to empower your healing sessions, crystals, and stones. These symbols can also be used to clear items, to send Reiki long distance, and much more. For example, you can use the symbols to empower your shampoo to encourage hair growth, your beauty products to last longer, your shower to assist you with releasing negative emotions, your food to empower your body, your money to spread kindness—the possibilities are limitless.

Healing Yourself

The goal of daily self-Reiki is to support overall wellness and spiritual growth. Daily self-practice assists the body in addressing existing problems before they turn into something more serious. Think of daily Reiki practice as a regular meditation practice. Just as preventative maintenance on our automobiles keeps them running smoothly, preventative maintenance for our bodies ensures that they stay healthy and running at their peak. By staying in balance and addressing issues as they come up, we further open the door for spiritual awakening.

We begin healing ourselves by listening to our bodies and ensuring they receive what is needed to function properly. This includes plenty of water, healthy food, sunshine, Reiki, and sleep.

Most often, when we feel blocked, it is because we are actually dehydrated. If you want your energy to flow at its best—for personal Reiki, treating others, or working on your intuitive abilities—it is crucial that you stay hydrated.

I have included multiple hand positions for self-care in later chapters. These positions are very effective for regaining balance, realigning the chakras, and building personal energy. But remember, it is up to you to make self-care a priority. When you are stressed, dehydrated, sleep deprived, or ill, you will not function properly.

Healing Others

Giving and receiving Reiki, watching other people see firsthand the marvelous possibilities of this energy, is truly remarkable. Reiki can be used to ease other people's pain, discomfort, and anxiety. Reiki can also be instrumental in helping people through a spiritual or existential crisis.

It has been my experience that we should not treat people with pacemakers or implanted battery-powered electronics or medical devices. Also, when treating people who have stainless or titanium pins or bone replacements, the Reiki often causes the metal to heat up or become warm. This does not damage the metal, but it may make the client uncomfortable. You should fully discuss this as a possibility before agreeing on a session.

CHILDREN, PETS, AND EVERYONE ELSE

We briefly discussed treating children and animals, but who or what else can be treated with Reiki? Everything! We can treat our food, our herb garden, our vitamins, and our medication. Everything is made of energy and can be programmed with Reiki. (By default, everything is programmed by the energy around it or the intention people use when creating an item.) Knowing this, you can open your practice even more by treating your home, your bathwater, and the very planet you live on.

When treating a client, we usually complete a 60-minute session, but when treating plants or animals we may need to spend only 10 to 15 minutes to see results. Because Reiki works to address not only medical issues, such as pain, but also spiritual distress, it can produce remarkable results quickly.

People are not the only ones to feel stress, anxiety, or fear. Consider how helpful Reiki could be to your children, pets, and plants in stressful situations. Even a spot treatment before a doctor's visit or long car ride can help immensely. This energy works to promote a deep sense of peace and acceptance.

Regular treatment sessions can also assist individuals in finding their way as their spiritual gifts and abilities come forward.

HEALING MULTIPLE PEOPLE

With Reiki, it is possible to heal multiple people at once. There are a number of ways we can facilitate this healing, from group Reiki sessions to long-distance methods. Although a person is more likely to have a spiritual experience during a one-to-one session, it is still possible to send Reiki to multiple people and witness their abilities grow as a group.

Setting Up a Session

Once you are attuned to Reiki energy, it is always with you and available for use. Setting up a Reiki session is easy as long as we remember a few important tips:

- Ensure your client is comfortable.
- Dedicate the correct amount of time to the session.
- Respect your client's privacy and boundaries.

We ensure clients are comfortable by giving them a safe place to experience Reiki, a space that is free from judgment and ensures privacy. As practitioners, we never know how someone will react to the Reiki energy. Someone sad or depressed may cry throughout the entire session or end up laughing. The energy conveys the experience the client needs. It is up to the practitioner to let clients know that they are in a safe, nonjudgmental, healing space.

If you are seeing clients in your home, create a private space away from other family members. If possible, make the space free from distractions, like sounds from the television or cooking smells. You may want to dim the lights, play soothing music, light incense, or diffuse essential oils.

No matter the setting, ensure your clients are comfortable by answering any and all questions they have about Reiki. Some folks will be very new to energy healing and could be nervous or anxious about the treatment. Take your time and answer their questions to the best of your ability. The more honest and forthcoming you are, the better. Remember, we never diagnose or tell clients to stop taking their medications.

Also, never promise clients certain results. It is important that the client knows the Reiki will do what it does and that this has very little to do with the wishes of the practitioner or client. This intelligent energy works to balance the physical, mental, emotional, and spiritual essence in a way that best fits the individual.

Create Space for Reiki

One of the coolest things about Reiki is it is self-contained and portable. Once you are attuned to Reiki energy, it is always with you. Reiki requires no machinery or special equipment, and it can be called on at any time, in any situation.

Although the ideal session would be performed in a soothing, peaceful room on a massage table with tranquil music playing in the background, this isn't always possible. Reiki can be done anywhere and most often is. We can do a mini session at home before job interviews, in our parked cars before we head home from the dentist, or at the kitchen table to help manage pain levels. Reiki will work as a spot treatment for common, everyday issues as well as more complex emotional problems. We create space for Reiki by practicing and intentionally tapping into this profound energy. Usually Reiki is just as intense in one's living room as it is in a hospital or clinical setting.

FACILITATING SPIRITUAL EXPERIENCES

Just performing Reiki can be a spiritual experience. While Reiki promotes physical wellness, it is also a natural catharsis for purging toxic trauma, negative energy, or outdated beliefs. By embracing who you are and learning to let go of the past, it is easy to become more empowered and authentic.

Reiki is inherently spiritual in nature and can activate latent intuitive abilities, as well as strengthen your craft. This wondrous energy strengthens our connection to Spirit, promotes self-awareness, and empowers us to make better decisions and end bad habits.

In the following chapter, you will learn how you can include Reiki in your day-to-day life to empower yourself and grow spiritually.

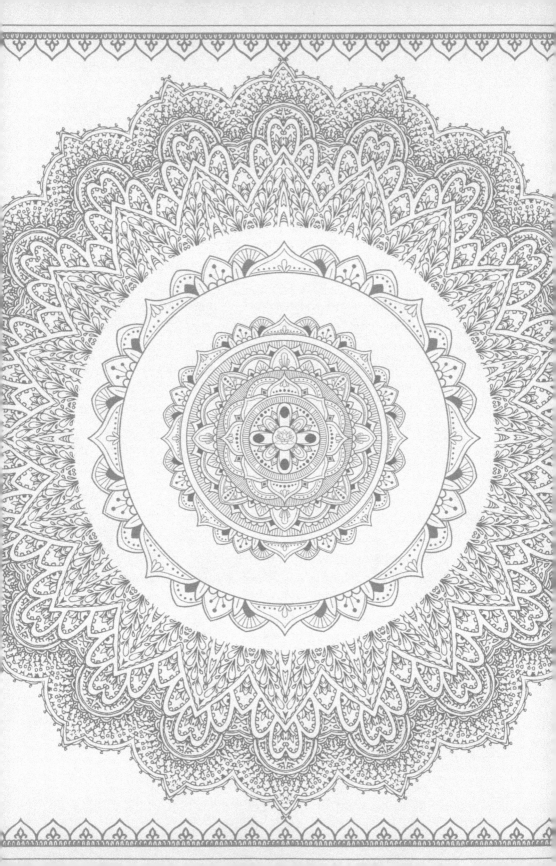

Chapter 3
Spiritual Reiki

Now that you have a better idea of the spectacular possibilities of working with Reiki, you may be wondering how you can apply it to your daily spiritual practice. The possibilities seem endless, but where do you begin? Also, it is normal to be curious about possible side effects or challenges associated with a spiritual awakening. Let's look deeper into what you can expect and discuss what a psychic transformation, or awakening, looks like and what challenges it may bring into your everyday life.

What Counts as a Spiritual Experience?

When we begin discussing spiritual experiences, the water can muddy quickly, as everyone has their own experiences and values.

Anything can be spiritual when we are in the flow of divine energy. Taoists consider everything to be part of the Tao. It is everywhere and almost impossible to understand because it is everything. To be present in the flow of this energy is to be 100 percent in the moment, totally alive and functioning, not fearing the future, ruminating on the past, or being distracted by the present. When we are in this flow, we experience divine synchronicity, like when you look at the clock and it's 11:11 or when you felt led to read this book. We understand nothing happens by chance or accident. We also stop second-guessing ourselves and understand that we are working with the Universe. We are in alignment with ourselves and our full potential. Life is effortless and easy again.

So that being said, what counts as a spiritual experience? There are many types and degrees of spiritual experiences. For some folks, a spiritual experience is witnessing something unexplainable, like a strange light in the sky. For other people, it is channeling a deceased loved one.

Some experiences come unasked for; others happen because we have set the stage with meditation, study, and intention. Once you begin to notice these episodes, you will see they have always been happening around you but perhaps in the background. But now, by tapping into Reiki, you see life with fresh eyes. By setting intentions and with the help of Reiki, you can bring more of these situations forward.

When we have a spiritual experience, we may be left feeling overwhelmed. As we become more used to this type of encounter, our reaction will change. We will begin to feel a deep connection to everything around us as we understand that anything is possible.

When we experience the spiritual side of life, we touch its mystery. We feel the awe of life around us and move from day-to-day drudgery to fascination. We can laugh at what we once feared and understand nothing is what we once thought it was. We are free to make our own choices based on awe rather than fear.

In this state, we let go of ego and worry. We move into the flow of intuitive knowing. We know that worry is pointless because we are able to draw anything we need to us. We know that anger is useless because nothing is actually aimed at us personally. This understanding frees us to step into compassion for others as well as ourselves.

We are then free to experience life on a deeper level. We notice changes in sunlight, sound, and even the texture of air on our skin. Our senses open and blossom, showing us that there is so much more to life and that WE are capable of so much more. What was once unimaginable, such as feeling new life in seedlings or knowing when someone will text, is now possible. We pull back the curtain and witness there are so many mysteries out there to be discovered. We find our zest for life.

Spiritual experiences lift you up and allow you to connect not only with yourself but also with the divine. The more you are in this flow, the more you realize you have and have always had amazing healing and intuitive powers. Spiritual experiences are the key that unlocks your ability to see yourself for the amazing being you truly are.

In later chapters we will discuss specific techniques to open your channels with Reiki. But for now, know you are right where the Universe wants you to be.

IT'S DIFFERENT FOR EVERYONE

Let me share one big truth with you: Everyone has spiritual gifts and abilities. Some people are aware of their gifts, while others attribute them to luck, instinct, or chance. Some people wish to close that part of themselves off or shut down these experiences altogether. If you are reading this book, that probably isn't you, but nonetheless, this is a safe, nonjudgmental space. There is no right or wrong approach to living with your abilities.

While Reiki is a great way to figure out what intuitive abilities you have, it can also level up the gifts you are already aware of and use. Reiki creates a safe and healthy space for exploring and nurturing your individual and unique abilities.

Hopefully, after taking Reiki classes you have met other like-minded people and are now part of a thriving psychic/spiritual community. We aren't in a race or competition in this community. We recognize that all gifts have merit and purpose. Everyone is important and everyone has something of value to contribute.

If, for example, you are an empath, then it is likely you started this adventure feeling more like your abilities were actually a curse, not a talent or a gift at all. But with Reiki, dedication, and practice, you will see you are blessed to have these abilities. There are, in fact, no bad or lesser abilities or gifts, which is why we never judge or compare ourselves to others. Working with Reiki, you can attain a new level of proficiency and understanding. You can shift from being at the mercy of your ability to learning how to use it to help others and make a positive impact on the world.

Know that your spiritual journey is as individual as you are. Our souls are here to grow, evolve, and learn. With a dedicated spiritual practice that includes Reiki, this journey becomes much easier.

A Natural Fit

Reiki is a natural, energy-healing modality that easily fits into your spiritual and wellness practice. Although Reiki is a subtle, gentle energy, it can have a big impact on your life. Often, when we are experiencing a problem, we see only the symptoms, but Reiki works on healing the underlying issue, even if we are unaware of the root cause. Reiki goes where it is most needed and facilitates a deep personal healing on many levels. Reiki can do no harm. Only good can come from practicing Reiki.

With the gift of Reiki, we can come back into balance. This energy works on body, mind, and spirit to help you regain your equilibrium and become a clearer, healthier version of yourself. As we move back into balance, life changes. We feel better psychically, and we are more emotionally centered and better able to handle day-to-day life. But Reiki also assists us on a much deeper level, clearing energy channels, replenishing the body, and allowing us to connect with our intuition and higher selves.

Here are some ways the benefits of Reiki may manifest:

- Being more mindful and present
- Being authentic in our dealings with others
- Being more accepting of life lessons
- Becoming more empathetic
- Stepping into the flow of manifestation
- Sensing and experiencing energy on a new level
- Boosting your psychic abilities
- Regaining your love of life

This transformation happens because all that energy that was once directed to just keeping us going can now be used more efficiently. Reiki, while not replacing conventional medical care, is a great addition to your spiritual and wellness practice.

HEALING IS A SPIRITUAL PRACTICE

Intuitives are naturally drawn to healing. While you may not be fully capable of expressing it, as an intuitive, you know that there is much more to life than the average person sees. Reiki could be the missing piece you have been searching for.

Intuitives naturally want to help others and the planet. They care about animals, crystals, and Mother Nature in a deep and loving way. If you're an intuitive, Reiki can aid your practice in ways you never expected. For example, checking into Reiki before yoga, crystal healing, or any type of energy practice will increase your results dramatically. We often witness this high-powered energy evoke an almost magical healing process.

Reiki is easily combined with other spiritual practices you may already have in place, empowering them and taking you deeper into the divine.

When we step into a mindful state with Reiki, even mundane tasks can become spiritual and healing in nature. Walking in the woods, eating a healthy meal, or spending time making art can lead to spiritual insights as this vibrant and calming energy permeates all you do.

Although Reiki is not faith-based and it works whether you believe in it or not, it is a very spiritual and nourishing energy.

REIKI OPENS YOU UP TO SPIRITUAL EXPERIENCES

Reiki can easily facilitate a spiritual awakening in the practitioner or client. If you have always felt different or connected to the spiritual world, Reiki (and some of the other practices we will discuss in this book) will assist you in furthering your spiritual knowledge and experiences.

As Reiki rebalances your chakras and energy centers, it opens you up to an entire new world of energy and experiences. No matter what other energy practices or spiritual crafts you perform, Reiki will empower and amplify your experience.

Reiki helps you balance your own energy and hold more of the higher vibrational energy needed to connect with higher realms. Illness, pain, and emotional upheaval are usually associated with a lower or unbalanced energy vibration. (Energy may even be blocked in the chakras.) The healer taps into Reiki and brings in a higher energy frequency that will raise the vibration of the client. For instance, we often observe that meditation, yoga, and mediumship become much easier with the support of Reiki. Your mind slows down and you have more control over your thoughts, allowing you to get out of your own head and listen to the divine.

It's Not Always What You'd Think

You may think that being spiritual is all about working with crystal balls, being instructed by otherworldly guides, or having heart-stopping visions, but actually, almost everyone has intuitive abilities. Most people don't even notice their gifts because they use them every day. Everyone is a little bit psychic, and although this energy can be subtle, it is very real. This energy manifests differently from person to person, but it is there. For instance, some folks are natural empaths and can feel the emotions of others. These folks may do this without even realizing what they are doing. They may not even consider it special or unique. Or you might consider yourself a bit witchy because odd things manifest in your life just because you think about them, or you could be experiencing synchronicity, like seeing 11:11 showing up around you. These abilities and others generally become clearer and make more sense after a Reiki attunement. New abilities and other gifts you never paid any attention to or even dismissed also increase. I was born with psychic abilities, but there was no instruction book, so for many years I drifted around looking for answers that just weren't there. Reiki was the missing piece that helped me understand my abilities. Not only did Reiki help me find a use for them, but my journey with this subtle energy also empowered me on many different levels as it increased my gifts.

You Might Experience . . .

You might be experiencing intuitive abilities while reading this book. Most people attuned to Reiki will feel a tingle just reading this. That is just one way spiritual abilities can manifest, but you could experience synchronicity as showing up at the right time and place to be offered a new job, or your inner guidance could become much louder after you become attuned to Reiki. Spiritual abilities can show up in many ways and take many different forms. Reiki might affect your abilities by empowering and strengthening them or by making them more intense. Let's briefly go over some of the more common abilities.

INTUITIVE ABILITIES

Intuitive abilities are often what most people think of when they hear the term *psychic*. Intuitive abilities usually manifest as a gut feeling or inner knowing, but they can also be classified as clairsentience, which means "clear feeling."

Intuitive abilities can develop over time and through various spiritual practices, such as Reiki. They are really very common and can often be so subtle that we overlook them. When you begin working with Reiki, you will feel more of everything, including more about the future, people, animals, and places. Reiki opens the door to stronger intuitive abilities and brings a better understanding of your gifts. Reiki clears up some of the mystery that often surrounds psychic experiences. Soon, you will be able to use your gifts with confidence and ease.

EMPATHY

Empaths and highly sensitive people are very common. Through practicing Reiki regularly, you may experience a profound heart chakra opening or healing that can unlock these powers, leading to latent abilities appearing or growing. As this ability manifests, it may take the form of intuitively knowing what other people are feeling or thinking. It also could manifest as knowing the mental state of your friends or family, even if they are across town or farther away. Most empaths experience a deepening of their abilities through Reiki. They may suddenly be able to feel the emotions of animals or connect with the crystal kingdom on a whole new level. Experiencing the feelings of others may present a challenge at first, but with patience, practice, and training, you will learn how to separate your own feelings from the emotions of others and use your talents to help others. Reiki can help you become more aware of the need for personal boundaries and self-care.

PSYCHIC ABILITIES

Reiki strengthens the body, mind, and energy field of all it touches. One of the side effects of this is the practitioner will see an increase in psychic abilities. Although this increase can vary from person to person, generally Reiki amplifies one's ability to hold both stronger energy and more energy. This increase of energy can often manifest as an overall increase in one's psychic abilities, as well as better overall health and clearer mental capacities.

We often see known psychic abilities, such as clairvoyance (clear seeing), clairaudience (clear hearing), and clairsentience (clear feeling), becoming stronger and easier to control, as well as new, unknown abilities manifesting. For instance, clairvoyance may develop suddenly and manifest as knowing when someone is thinking about you and is about to text or call. Clairaudience often manifests as suddenly having improved hearing. You may be very sensitive to sounds and be able to hear whispered conversations some distance away. Clairsentience often appears as feeling the emotions of people around you or feeling what has happened in a room before you enter.

Experiencing psychic abilities can be challenging if you do not know or understand what is happening, which is another reason to have a teacher you can talk with. Although these new gifts might be challenging at first, regular self-Reiki and self-care will help you integrate them into your everyday life.

VISIONS

It is not uncommon for Reiki masters as well as Reiki clients to report seeing colors, symbols, or visions during a session. Visions usually manifest through the third eye chakra, but they can also be experienced as objects or people suddenly presenting themselves in the physical space around you.

Some folks see people, animals, guides, or angels, while others see spirits, ghosts, ascended masters, and elementals. Generally, it is better to see what's there than to be blind to it, although seeing can be a challenge, especially in the beginning. As you become accustomed to seeing, you will also learn that most of what is portrayed in novels and television shows is exaggerated or completely wrong. We share space with many beings; most pay us no notice at all. For example, let's say you have a small green space in front of your home, and on this space there is a small ant colony. You pass by it every time you leave and enter your home. Do you know the names or habits of the ants? Do you interact with the ants? Probably not. It is the same with most of our interactions with spirits. So, while seeing other beings may be unnerving in the beginning, you will learn that most of what you are seeing is no more harmful than a colony of ants.

One of the more odd side effects of working with Reiki is we are less likely to see illusions. For example, we are less likely to see heat patches rising from roads in the summer in hot climates and are less likely to be tricked by optical illusions. Almost everyone perceives these mirage images, but after being attuned to Reiki and working with it, you will no longer see these types of mirages or optical illusions.

When seeing or sensing any new energy, we must remain calm and not react or overreact. Staying calm may take practice, especially when you see energy take shape in a room around people. But with practice, you will learn to discern what is physical and what is from other realms.

MEDIUMSHIP

Many, but not all Reiki masters are also mediums. A medium isn't the same as a psychic, but some psychics are also mediums, and many people are both. Mediums connect with loved ones in spirit form and pass along messages to specific individuals. Psychics, on the other hand, may read energy, see visions, intuitively know information, or work with their own guides to gather information. It is fairly common to see apparitions or deceased family members when undergoing an attunement or even during a Reiki session. If a person's natural talent is clairvoyance, then Reiki may open up this gift.

With proactive exercise and training, this talent often becomes something that one can tap into at will, allowing you to talk to discarnate entities, ancestors, and spirits. These entities could be other spiritual beings, deceased beings, angels, ascended masters, or other dimensional beings. Each brings with it its own challenge.

Using Reiki as your foundation, and with proper training, you can obtain more levels of mediumship. This ability can, of course, be a challenge in everyday life until it is mastered.

DREAMS

Vivid and evocative dreams usually accompany a Reiki attunement. Dreams can also manifest after a Reiki treatment, as your chakras move into alignment and you heal. Often Reiki masters report remembering vivid, lucid dreams like never before. It is also common to remember dreams of working with guides and angels, and to attend spiritual night school on a regular basis. If dreaming is your gift, Reiki will increase and empower it. This increased ability could manifest as accessing more realms, learning from extra-dimensional beings, or bringing back more information from dreaming.

You may also find that Reiki magnifies your clairvoyant and clairsentient abilities as you remember more and more information gained from lucid dreaming. Lucid dreaming is a fascinating discipline based on the ability to wake up in dreams and know that you are dreaming. The lucid dreamer is then able to manipulate the dream state to gather information, complete tasks, heal, and interact on different planes with other beings. Signs this ability is awakening can often be felt as a pressure on the top of the head or crown chakra, as well as an itchy sensation in the middle of the forehead around the sixth chakra.

Astral projection, also called astral travel, describes an intentional out-of-body experience that allows the soul or consciousness to leave the physical body. The consciousness can then travel away from the physical body. Out-of-body experiences are also common after working with Reiki.

SEEING AURAS

Most of my students have reported that after the initial attunement, they begin to see everything around them differently. Colors are much brighter than before, and they can discern an outline around people and animals that was not visible before. This subtle shift in perception is brought on by aligning and opening the sixth chakra with Reiki.

Most Reiki schools teach the technique for seeing auras in the level one class. After the initial attunement, you may notice that your third eye chakra may itch or feel much more sensitive than before, a signal that it is opening up.

While seeing auras might sound challenging, it is something you can easily get used to and it will become normal soon.

PSYCHIC OR MEDICAL INTUITIVE

Since I often treat clients with physical problems, Reiki allows me to intuitively know or hear medical situations they may be experiencing. Although we never diagnose, understanding that a person is in a great deal of pain or is having joint issues, for example, can be helpful in discussing the client's overall condition. This can be a challenge when people are surprised that you are aware of things they have not shared yet, but over time you learn how best to use this ability.

NO MATTER WHAT TYPE

No matter what gifts or combination of abilities manifest, know that they are perfectly normal. We all have our own paths to follow, and you are not competing against other people. Each of us is working on healing and growing into our own skills. Your abilities may manifest in completely different ways or at a different rate, and that's okay.

Over time, you will master these gifts and make room for more abilities to flourish. You can use Reiki to further tap into and develop these hidden abilities as you grow on your spiritual path.

Auras

Auras are often seen as an outline of color or colors moving around a person or object. They can be bright or soft, static or swirling, intense or very subtle. You will learn in the Reiki level one class how to see auras around people, animals, and plants. You may also see auras if your third eye chakra is open and functioning. Reiki will intensify this ability, and you may easily see auras without concentration or much practice. An aura can change based on a person's mental, emotional, and physical health as well as emotional state. Intense emotions, chronic pain, and general health will impact the vitality of the color as well as the condition of the aura. Some people have more of an outline following the curves of the body, while others have more of an egg or oval shape of light glowing or surrounding them. Stress, worry, medication, addiction, intense emotions, spiritual practices, physical health, and levels of creativity may affect a person's aura. A creative person, for example, may have a patch of maroon or orange color swirling in a mix of other colors, while an ill person may have gaps or what look like holes in the energy field. Usually, we see a very subtle band of color or colors swirling around clients when we are treating them with Reiki, but what practitioners see also depends on their gifts.

SPIRITUAL GUIDES

Many cultures believe that we are always in contact with unseen spirits, ancestors, or guides. Some people call these our guardian angels, while others say they are spirits of our ancestors. I personally believe it can be either or even both. We also can have more than one guide or angel. Some come and go, assisting us through difficult spots in our life, while others are a more long-term guiding force.

Our ability to contact these guides often manifests after a Reiki attunement. Some people hear a voice in their mind and begin to see shapes, outlines, or shadows of people, while others hear an external voice speaking, as if someone were in the room with them. *Your guide will never tell you to hurt yourself or harm anyone else. Your guide will not yell at, coax, or bully you.* Negative voices are more likely your own internal turmoil and a manifestation of past trauma. Guides are subtle, loving, often overlooked voices that praise and encourage us. They offer wisdom and advice that allows us to grow and flourish, not suffer or harm ourselves.

Guides can manifest as animals, people from our past who have passed on, or ascended masters. They can communicate with us also through synchronicity, such as seeing 11:11 or other repeating numbers constantly. (Try keeping your journal handy and writing down what happens around the time you see 11:11 or 3:33.) Guides also send us messages through pictures, television, or music. You may be thinking about a problem and suddenly a song comes over the radio that holds the perfect answer to the dilemma. This experience could be accompanied by a cold shiver or goose bumps, announcing your guide is present. Look for anomalies around you and journal what you find. The more you become aware, the more you will notice your guides are constantly in contact.

Guides also communicate to us through dreams. For instance, in a dream, you may meet someone that you never actually fully see. This person is always beside you, but you cannot see the person's face or body type. But the guide proves helpful and wise in the course of the dream. You may enjoy the person's camaraderie, feel at ease, and see the same person in multiple dreams. The guide usually feels very familiar, too, like a long-lost friend.

You may have other types of encounters with guides by using tools such as tarot or oracle cards. Many people also work with their guides by using a pendulum for communication. However you approach working with spirit guides, always remember that you have the final say and do not ever have to follow their advice blindly. They are there to guide you, not control you.

Spiritual and Emotional Healing

At its core, Reiki is intended to be a self-healing modality. When we commit to a daily practice of Reiki, we begin to notice our own trauma and personal issues coming up to be addressed and healed. Once we sort out these issues and release the anger, guilt, and pain, we no longer feel the need to self-medicate or engage in self-sabotaging behaviors.

In this healthier state, our spiritual abilities grow and flourish. The key is being open to both the personal healing and the spiritual aspect of Reiki. To be a better healer, you have to stop running from your own pain and work through it.

By healing ourselves, we help heal others. Our empathy and compassion grow, as does our emotional maturity, making us better able to help others and support them on their own spiritual journeys.

BENEFITS TO PRACTITIONER AND CLIENT

Increased spiritual abilities are not limited solely to practitioners; clients frequently experience major energy shifts after a session. Often clients report seeing colors, symbols, or visions during a Reiki session. They regularly report feeling the energy working directly on their bodies as a tingle or chill. The energy can also be felt as a pressure-like or magnetic sensation or even as a touch while doing non-touch Reiki.

While the energy works on the physical body, it also improves the energy flow of the chakras, removing emotional blocks and revitalizing the energy body. This improvement often results in clients becoming more intuitive, accessing hidden abilities, and tapping into their own spirituality. New abilities, as well as other heightened senses, may surface. Reiki has so many wonderful benefits for both the practitioner and the client.

Who Needs Spiritual Healing?

Everyone can benefit from spiritual healing. While it is easy to assume only people going through emotional upheaval need this healing, in fact we all need it. Many people ignore their spiritual lives in favor of just getting through the day, and who can blame them? Life can be tough, but when we address our personal pain and suffering, life can dramatically change.

It is common for spiritual awakenings to take place after a personal loss or major life event. This happens because we are (naturally) so devastated by these events that we cannot move forward until some spiritual healing takes place. As I can attest, Reiki can be very helpful for people going through grief or loss. Taking time for personal sessions or meditating with Reiki can give much-needed relief from a churning, overwrought mind and the emotional agony surrounding these events. Reiki also works on moving the heavy and stagnant energy of the trauma off the physical and emotional bodies, allowing for healing on many levels.

Regardless of what you are going through, be it a major upheaval or just trying to find your way, Reiki can help. We are not meant to just survive this life; we are meant to thrive. We are meant to lead a life of wonder, growth, and delight, and the key to this is personal healing. Deep and meaningful personal growth cannot happen until we address our own issues.

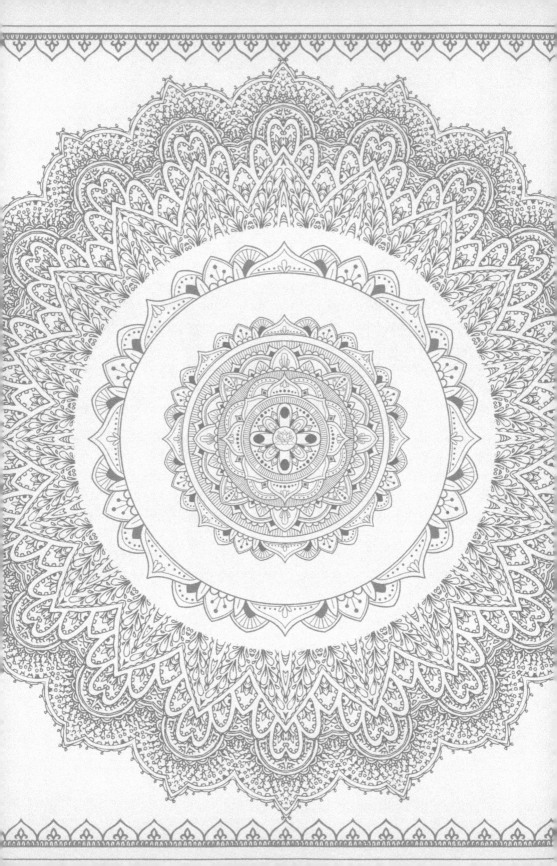

Chapter 4

Tapping Into Your Spiritual Abilities

In this chapter, we will go deeper into tapping into your spiritual gifts. There are many ways Reiki can help you awaken and grow intuitive abilities. Building a spiritual practice you can stick with is key. Resist the urge to measure your gifts against others—all spiritual abilities have merit, and all come in their own time. Very few people just wake up one day with the ability to read minds or hear their guides. It takes time and commitment to build a solid practice. Your routine should make you happy and empowered so that you stick with it. Practice leads to results. Commit to these exercises, practices, and Reiki to begin awakening your true abilities.

Keep Your Third Eye Open

You may know what your spiritual abilities are, or you may be searching for them. One common yet subtle ability many people take for granted is clairvoyance. This ability begins with a healthy third eye chakra and is key in true seeing. Clairvoyant abilities usually begin to manifest in small, subtle ways. Here are some examples:

- Sensing someone's about to call or text you
- Knowing that perfect sweater you wanted is going to be on sale this week
- Being aware that another car is about to cut you off in traffic

- Knowing when a package is being delivered to your home
- Having strange yet prophetic dreams of the future

Physically, you may notice a tingle in the middle of your forehead as the third eye chakra becomes active. You may also notice colors are more intense and vibrant.

Reiki energy flows directly to the third eye chakra to remove blocks and rebalance this energy center. When it is healthy and open, it will allow you to experience your world very differently.

BE OPEN AND RECEPTIVE

You probably have noticed odd things happening in the past and either ignored or forgot them. This is common, because with everything going on in life, we tend to forget or ignore what we can't readily explain. Here are a few simple tips to help you become more receptive to your intuitive and spiritual abilities:

Journal. Keep a journal with you or use your phone and take notes as things happen. Our minds have a way of making us forget things they cannot explain. You are much more intuitive than you know, and there is proof in your everyday life. By keeping a journal and revisiting it at least weekly, you will soon see this.

Be more open. Often when we feel something (or someone) is "off," we usually dismiss it as being paranoid or judgmental. Next time this happens, before you dismiss this thought, ask yourself where it is coming from. Do you have past experiences with these types of situations, making this a logical assumption, or is it something else? If not, then where is this feeling coming from? Note the feeling and any bodily sensations (like a headache or upset stomach). Then pay attention as the situation plays out. Were you right from the beginning?

Ask for signs. Take a moment to calm your mind, center yourself, and ask your guide to show you a sign that you can understand, such as finding a feather, hearing a name suddenly repeated over and over, or a cold shiver running down your arm.

Let go. Often we attempt to micromanage everything, leaving little room for us to notice the magic around us. By meditating and learning to leave room for our guides and spiritual abilities to flourish, we invite growth and can see the divine in everyday life.

Quiet the mind. By learning to quiet the mind, we make room to hear. Usually spirit guides, like our own intuition, speak softly and can be very hard to hear in an overwhelmed, monkey-mind state. By clearing our minds, we can hear what is always there. One quick way to clear your mind is to do a brain dump—grab a piece of paper and write out everything that you are thinking. By putting your thoughts on paper, you no longer have to think over details or problems. You can then sit quietly and invite your guide to speak with you.

INVITE SPIRITUAL EXPERIENCES

During a Reiki session, you can invite spiritual experiences simply by allowing them space to unfold. Going into a session without preconceived ideas or trying to micromanage the energy will allow ample space for these experiences to come forward in their own way.

Also, the cleaner the container (your body), the less Reiki is used to rebalance your system and the more it can work on empowering your abilities. Once your health improves, energy can be channeled into higher vibrational experiences and intuitive gifts. Allowing your abilities to unfold in their own way and shape means learning to trust the experience and stop second-guessing yourself.

Reiki and Intuitive Abilities

We all have intuitive abilities, and Reiki can directly affect how these gifts manifest in our lives. Usually after a level one Reiki attunement, new spiritual abilities awaken and manifest. These abilities may be subtle, such as knowing what food you should eat and what to avoid, or stronger, like having physical reactions to other people's emotions and personal energy. You may be able to pick up much more information from a card reading or connect with crystals on a much deeper level. As the Reiki moves through your energy system removing blocks from your chakras, you could experience many different intuitive abilities, ranging from very subtle to life changing.

TAP INTO YOUR GIFTS

Now that you have identified some of your spiritual gifts, you can learn to tap into them at will. It is easy to tap into your spiritual gifts when you are in balance. Reiki also flows easier when we are in a relaxed, balanced state. Less energy is used healing our bodies when we are healthy and relaxed. Freeing up energy to empower your abilities is an important step in accessing your gifts. If you want to fully tap into and harness your own abilities, you should begin by working on yourself:

- Work on healing your own personal trauma.
- Begin a daily journal practice.
- Commit to focused movement (such as yoga, belly dance, or tai chi) to move stuck energy.
- Be present (work on mindfulness).
- Stop smoking.
- Commit to a daily meditation practice.
- Give up harmful habits and stop using recreational drugs.
- Stop consuming junk/processed food.
- Consider following a plant-based diet, a vegan lifestyle, or eating as clean as possible.
- Commit fully to a healing self-care routine.

A Welcoming Environment

We can create a clean, inviting environment to welcome spiritual experiences. Setting the stage and clearing the way expresses our intentions around Reiki and healing. Let go of clutter, rubbish, and personal judgment. Instead, create a warm, loving space. Pick an area of your home or garden as your personal space. This can be an area of your bedroom or a cozy, private corner of your garden. Keep the area clean and in good repair. Decorate your space with things you love, such as crystals, family mementos, plants, chakra stones, candles, magical items, and other meaningful collections. Make this area a place you want to spend time in and use it for meditation and spiritual craft work. Most people do both physical and energetic cleaning before they begin energy work. Clear yourself and your space of all clutter, mental and physical. Use sage smoke, burn incense, or diffuse essential oils to cleanse yourself and the area. You can also take a salt bath before you begin your practice. We create a welcoming spiritual environment by being focused and 100 percent present. Meditate, relax, and calm yourself. Spirit—or the divine or sense of magic—is always with you, but by making space in your life to talk and listen, you open yourself up to an entirely new experience. If you feel you cannot meditate because your mind will not settle down, try this: Grab your favorite stone or crystal and sit comfortably on the floor. Close your eyes and softly chant the name of the Reiki power symbol for three to five minutes. This practice will further your connection to Reiki, calm your mind, and energize your body.

Tuning in to your gifts is not about buying into trends, owning the correct crystal, or doing the perfect yoga posture. It's about cleaning your container (your body and mind) and connecting to your higher self in your own way. When you do, you will expand your consciousness and tap into your spiritual gifts with ease and grace.

SPIRITUAL AWAKENINGS

Reiki can be the core of your spiritual practice, and it often initiates a deep, internal spiritual awakening in clients as well as practitioners. This awakening may appear first as a healing crisis, such as suddenly having unexplainable flu-like symptoms (including aches and pains) that randomly come and go. It may also manifest as old trauma surfacing, even though you are sure you have let it go or forgotten the experience. You may experience bouts of fatigue, dizziness, ringing in the ears, or extreme sensitivity to weather, foods, or sounds. You may also experience a period of release as you let go of past issues, such as heartbreak or emotional pain associated with grief or loss. This release can be radical forgiveness or popcorn epiphanies that happen one right after the other as you experience sudden insights regarding your life choices. As this healing happens, a huge spiritual shift occurs. Suddenly you may care less about what people think of you and more about being authentic, for example.

Your life begins to change as you make decisions based on what's right for you and not what other people are doing or societal norms. You may find, for instance, that you are more sensitive to drama and can no longer watch the news or even some popular dramatic television programs. Your taste in music may also change as you understand that listening to and singing along with violent or negative lyrics is not attracting the experiences you want. You may no longer like the same types of food, preferring a healthier, balanced diet over fast food. It is also common to suddenly and effortlessly stop an addiction when you experience a spiritual awakening.

Some spiritual awakenings hit like a ton of bricks and may include integrating deep lessons and a detox period. Other times, they are subtle and accompany a new understanding of your life's purpose and are intensely freeing and uplifting.

ATTUNEMENTS AND DEVELOPING GIFTS

As we have already discussed, undergoing a Reiki attunement can be a profound healing and spiritual experience. The attunement ceremony may also jump-start latent abilities or open the door for new gifts.

Reiki attunements clear, empower, and open the crown, third eye, heart, and palm chakras, allowing energy to flow freely through these powerful energy centers. The hands become much more sensitive. The crown, third eye, and heart become more open to higher vibrations, and we are better equipped to process these new sensations. We begin collecting information from these newly opened chakras as our abilities unfold in unimaginable ways.

The attunement allows Reiki to flow freely through the body 24 hours a day, aligning, healing, and empowering. As the body comes back into balance, the energy opens and empowers psychic gifts. The Reiki also assists the practitioner in coming to terms with these changes, enabling the practitioner to understand and assimilate the weight of these gifts. Past fears may be released, and self-judgment or competition may no longer be an issue. We embrace who we are and our developing gifts.

DEVELOPING YOURSELF

To develop your abilities, you will need to clear distractions and commit to working on yourself. This may be somewhat challenging, but the rewards far outweigh the minor inconvenience of taking better care of yourself.

Meditate. Meditation and learning to quiet your mind help immensely in developing your abilities. Meditation also strengthens your concentration and develops your focus, helping you distinguish your thoughts and ego from spiritual messages.

Intuitive Experiences While Healing

Intuitive experiences vary from practitioner to practitioner, but it is common to see colors or even full visions while performing a healing session. As you clear your mind and allow the Reiki to flow through you (remember we never direct the energy—it goes where it is needed), you may see glimpses of events related to the client or issues the client is struggling with. Your chakras may buzz or tingle as the energy moves from you to the client, and you may feel very happy and content. You may also intuitively know where the client is having pain or feel an emotion the client is struggling with. Your angels or spirit guides may tell you what issues or medical conditions the client is suffering from. It is not uncommon to smell roses or other pleasant scents in the room during a session, especially when guides are present. Some people see symbols, swirling colors, golden light, or past lives during sessions. The practitioner may also notice that heart chakra issues, for instance, require more energy than physical issues. Know that what happens is meant to happen. Reiki is intelligent energy that will direct the healing experience for the client's greater good, and we should give it ample space to flow. Most people feel very light and peaceful while performing Reiki, because every time a practitioner performs a Reiki session, the practitioner also receives a healing.

Practice. Make time daily to practice and learn more about your gifts. There are many ways you can further study and develop your abilities. Begin by writing out the experiences you have had and try to reproduce them. Work toward control and accuracy while still enjoying yourself.

Perform self-Reiki. One of the best ways to develop your spiritual abilities is by taking the time to practice self-Reiki every day. Giving yourself even a quick spot treatment that focuses on the major chakras is very beneficial. People often ask me how long an average self-Reiki session should last. Just as when we treat others, when we treat ourselves, the amount of time we spend Reiking the chakras should be determined by the flow of energy at each location. Don't rush through the process, but don't dismiss self-Reiki because you feel you do not have enough time either. Like with meditation, the times we need Reiki the most are often the moments we are most overwhelmed and stressed out.

Eliminate toxins from your body. So much energy is used in processing and eliminating toxins from the body that there isn't much left over for spiritual development. Eat healthy and give up toxic behaviors that drain your energy. Give your body space to heal and renew itself and watch how your abilities bloom.

Commit to an active self-care routine. Self-care is a term bounced around on social media all the time. We see posts of hair salon visits and lovely bathtubs filled with flowers and surrounded by candles and tumbled stones. While these things are nice, they're not accurate representations of self-care. Real self-care is more than artsy baths and getting your hair done. Going to the salon, like going to the gym, is maintenance because it requires active external energy. True self-care is about relaxing, de-stressing, and taking care of yourself. Self-care should include going deep inside and doing intrapersonal healing. There are many ways to do this, from therapy sessions to journaling, but the focus should be on healing and restoring, not on escaping.

HELPING OTHERS DEVELOP THEIR GIFTS

With Reiki, we can help others develop their spiritual abilities and gifts. If your clients or friends are interested in this side of Reiki, you can easily help them tap into their hidden gifts with regular healing sessions, chakra meditations, chanting, breath work, and many other practices.

Leading a relaxing, guided meditation after a Reiki session, for example, can allow people to tap into their gifts in a safe, inviting space. You can also help others tap into their abilities by connecting them with their spirit guides or discussing after a Reiki session what they saw in their mind's eye during that session.

Even just letting others know you have experiences and abilities in the areas they wish to grow in can be very empowering and helpful. Answering their questions and encouraging them to try their abilities in a safe, nonjudgmental space is also helpful. Having someone to work with can be a great way to begin this journey.

USING YOUR GIFTS RESPONSIBLY

Once your gifts begin to bloom, you may be caught in an ethical dilemma. For example, let's say you are at a restaurant having a nice dinner with your family. As the server comes to refill your drink, you suddenly feel that he has a very ill mother and she may not make it through the week. What should you do? Almost all of my students have experienced this ethical dilemma at one time or another. First, let's look at the circumstances and then the expected outcome if you use your gifts in this situation.

Energy is everywhere, all around us and connected to everything imaginable. Now that you are sensing energy and can read and interact with it, you may feel compelled to give messages to everyone. This isn't always the wisest course of action, though. Just because you know something doesn't mean you should act on it. Imagine you are driving down a freeway, and you begin to see billboards that advertise restaurants, BBQ places, motels, and so on. You are only going a short way and not planning on stopping to eat or stay the night. So this information, while helpful overall, isn't really meant for you. Picking up intuitive messages is just like this. You are picking up information that may not be meant for you. If you feel that you must deliver a message to someone, be mindful of the person's feelings. Ask yourself how you would feel if someone delivered such a message to you, especially unasked. Will this information be helpful to them? Also consider how you would react if someone delivered this message to you out of the blue. What if you were the server? How would you feel if someone blurted out your mother was going to die?

Also be prepared for a dubious, or even hostile, response. You could be scolded, mocked, or even threatened for delivering uninvited bad news.

The best way to use your gifts is to be mindful of other people's feelings. Perhaps you could hand them a business card to tell them that you practice Reiki and invite them for a session. By taking the time to talk with them, you open the door for them to ask questions or allow them to move on if they aren't interested. They may welcome your insights or be dismissive, but ultimately you created a safe space for them and allowed them to make the choice.

Furthering Your Spiritual Practice

How can you further your spiritual practice? You may already know that you have intuitive abilities or are an empath or a medium, but by incorporating Reiki into your practice, you can open the door to move beyond those gifts. After several Reiki sessions, you will likely notice an increase in your abilities, and after an attunement, they will expand and increase dramatically. You can also further spirituality in your daily life through ordinary, everyday activities, such as journaling, meditation, self-Reiki, and self-care. Compassion, being of service, and taking responsibility for your personal healing will empower you and initiate a deep healing. This healing can be the catalyst for your spiritual practice to change, grow, and develop into something more. Often at this point we see an increase in abilities in unexpected and dramatic ways. Working with teachers, taking spiritual classes, and helping others on their spiritual paths will further your spiritual practice.

TAKING CLASSES

People often ask me when the best time is to take a Reiki course. My answer is, "Now!" The present moment is always the best time to begin your journey into Reiki. If we wait, we will find excuses not to move forward on the healing path.

While learning more about healing or spiritual abilities may take you out of your comfort zone, it isn't as frightening as you may think. Reiki is actually easy to learn, and depending on the setting, it may trigger a huge personal healing and transformation, unlocking new spiritual abilities and empowering other gifts.

There are many classes that can help you better understand energy healing, the chakras, crystals, and how to grow your intuition. If you are feeling lost and overwhelmed, you can find me online at Serenity Reiki Clinic, and I will be happy to help you find your way.

So, if you are wondering when you should begin a spiritual class or take a Reiki course, don't wait!

FINDING A SPIRITUAL TEACHER

It is wise to talk to potential Reiki teachers before signing up for a class. Most of us love to talk about Reiki and will be more than happy to talk your ear off! Ask prospective teachers what type of Reiki they teach, how long they have been studying Reiki, and how long the classes are. Also find out what else is included in the class, how many students will be attending, and if you will receive a textbook or anything else.

Make sure you will receive an attunement, and ask questions about the format of the class. Will it be taught in person, online, or via pre-recorded video or audio? Ask the teacher to discuss the syllabus for the course and any other questions you have about Reiki. The teacher should be able to answer your questions and easily explain what is covered in the course.

You should also feel comfortable with the teacher. It's important that you feel you can ask questions and understand the phrases or terms the teacher uses. Briefly explain your personal spiritual practice to the prospective teacher and ask how they feel taking spiritual Reiki classes will enhance it. Some schools approach Reiki from different viewpoints. You should find a teacher that fits well with yours.

Ask prospective teachers how the attunement process will affect your spiritual awakening and what you should expect during and immediately following class. Look for clarity on these subjects as well as general knowledge. It is important that teachers understand their own spiritual practices, as well as how Reiki will affect others.

Important Things to Note When Looking for a Reiki Teacher/School:

- Ask all potential Reiki teachers how they feel about the spiritual side of Reiki and what experiences they have had personally.
- Ask teachers how they define spiritual Reiki and what you should expect in the course.
- Do not dismiss a teacher who is new to teaching. Ask all the teachers you speak with how they regularly work with clients and practice self-Reiki. This aspect is more important than how long they have been teaching.
- Almost all Reiki schools honor classes taught by other Reiki teachers, which means if you take a traditional level one class from a teacher in London and then move to Boston, you should find a traditional Reiki teacher that will honor your level one status and not make you repeat the level. When you speak with prospective teachers, ask them whether your previous training will be recognized.

- Similarly, most Reiki schools allow past students to sit in any Reiki class they have already attended and passed at that school as a refresher, free of charge. Ask if the school follows this rule.

Ask any questions you may have before signing up for class and embrace the experience!

Take Care of Yourself

Tapping into your spiritual abilities can be super exciting, but with it comes personal responsibilities. Responsibility isn't just about how we ethically use our abilities; it's also how we treat our bodies. Psychic fatigue is a common problem for most intuitives. When developing your spiritual abilities, you need to factor in more time for rest and self-care. Having a psychic hangover can feel like an alcohol-fueled hangover, minus the alcohol. You may feel that you were out too late, totally exhausted, and fatigued. Psychic fatigue could also include a terrible headache or hypersensitivity to light, sound, and smells. Normal sensations may overwhelm you and make you sick to your stomach. It is important to educate yourself on the best techniques to prevent these and other symptoms.

How do you cure a psychic hangover? It's best to begin a self-care routine now and avoid an energy hangover, but if you are suffering from these types of symptoms, Reiki can work wonders on easing your fatigue. After you are feeling better, review your actions to better understand what caused the fatigue. Were you working too long with tarot cards or practicing your intuitive abilities online too intensely? Or were you attempting to do a reading before you grounded and shielded yourself? (For more on grounding with Reiki, refer to the Reiki hand positions.) Could you be pushing yourself on too little sleep and not enough water? Were you spending hours around low-vibing friends, coworkers, or family members who were sucking your energy up?

Reiki is amazing at replenishing your energy, but you should treat your spiritual studies as you would anything else. When you are tired, take a break or quit for the day. Allow yourself time to recover before returning, and work on supporting your efforts with healthy self-care. This may mean getting enough sleep and eating healthy foods. Proper self-care is vital to healthy spiritual development.

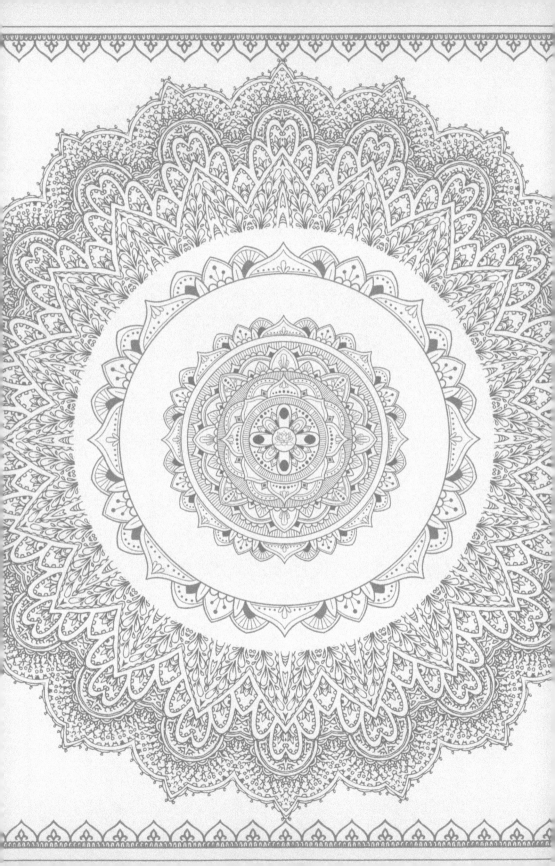

Chapter 5

Enhance Your Spiritual Practice

Reiki can be a wonderful and safe foundation for your spiritual practice. As you have already learned, Reiki works well in combination with other holistic and natural practices to facilitate deep physical, mental, and spiritual healing.

In this chapter, we will cover other spiritual practices that can be used to complement and enhance Reiki healing and grow your spiritual abilities.

Combinations and Complements

Reiki works amazingly well in tandem with other spiritual practices. It is safe, intelligent, unlimited energy that can do no harm. It will adapt and empower most practices and healing modalities and strengthen your connection to the divine.

Reiki is unlike other healing energies in that it does not take energy from the practitioner nor draw energy from the earth. Most traditional healing modalities use the life force energy of the practitioner. Some even transfer the illness or problem from the client's body to the practitioner's. Reiki is different in that it pulls in energy from all around us (what we call universal life force energy). The practitioner is never left depleted or ill after a treatment. In fact, because practitioners channel the energy through their bodies, they receive a healing session. The more you practice Reiki, the more you heal yourself as well.

If you are unsure about blending other practices with Reiki, you may safely use Reiki after any spiritual practice. It can restore and revitalize you after an intense workout, yoga session, or mystical experience.

An Inclusive Art

Reiki is adaptive and inclusive, which is why there are so many ways it can be modified to work with other modalities. At its heart, Reiki is an intelligent, safe, adaptive, and accommodating energy. You can implement this subtle yet dynamic energy in your healing arts practice and make it the foundation of your personal spiritual routine. Reiki should form the basis of your healing and spiritual system, as it lends itself to opening up many possibilities for you.

Reiki is suitable for fragile clients yet strong enough to blast through chakra blocks and reveal hidden abilities. Reiki adapts to the client's needs and works with other modalities to bring about the best overall results.

Reiki will change and enhance all your healing techniques. You will see immediate results in your yoga practice, as well as your crystal healing. Reiki can easily add power and direction to other modalities, giving them the energy they need to morph into a full spiritual practice.

CRYSTALS

Crystal energy can greatly complement your Reiki practice and vice versa. Although crystals and stones should not be a substitute for medical care, they can complement Reiki and all it brings.

If you are new to the crystal healing world, you may want to begin with inexpensive and easy-to-find crystals. Visit a store that sells crystals and see what calls to you. Allow yourself to be led by your intuition. Here are five great crystals to begin with:

> **Rose quartz** is the go-to stone for all matters of love but especially for self-love. If you are struggling with self-confidence or self-esteem, working with rose quartz can help you feel more empowered and confident. Meditate with or wear a piece of rose quartz that has been empowered with Reiki to help remove heart chakra blocks and restore energy levels.

Smoky quartz is a wonderful stone to work with to balance emotions and relieve tension, stress, anxiety, or panic attacks. Invoke Reiki and hold this stone in your dominant hand, sit quietly, and focus on your breathing. Soon you should feel more relaxed and at peace.

Malachite is a heart chakra stone that has many uses. It is wonderful for manifesting as well as for cleansing and removing negative, stuck energy blocks. When empowered with Reiki, this lovely stone is thought to fortify your aura, remove stale or stuck energy from its surroundings, and invite in positive energy.

Fluorite is believed to calm a troubled mind and promote relaxation and deeper, regenerative sleep. Wear fluorite to aid with focus and concentration and place a small, tumbled piece under your pillow to improve sleep and remember your dreams. Also, placing a piece of Reiki-empowered fluorite in your home is thought to offer energetic protection from unwanted spirts.

Black obsidian is an amazing grounding stone. If you have trouble staying focused or suffer from monkey mind, try wearing or carrying a small, Reiki-empowered piece of tumbled black obsidian. Black obsidian is also thought to be a strong psychic protection stone and can be placed inside your home's entryway to stop psychic attacks.

ESSENTIAL OILS

Essential oils work very well with Reiki. They can help enhance a client's overall relaxation experience and aid the healing process. I often diffuse essential oils during a session or add a drop of lavender to my natural coconut oil hand lotion before beginning a session. As my hands hover over the client's body, the client will smell the scents and relax further. There are many, many essential oils that work well with Reiki and have a myriad of uses, but if you are new to essential oils, I would suggest you begin with a few simple and inexpensive oils, such as lavender, sandalwood, and lemon.

Lavender: As mentioned above, I think the scent of lavender is very relaxing for most people. When we add this powerful oil to a Reiki session, the client can go into a deeper state of relaxation, tranquility, and peace.

Sandalwood: This amazing oil works well with Reiki. The deep, mysterious scent instills a deep calmness in most people. When paired with Reiki, it helps balance the lower three chakras.

Lemon: When lemon essential oil is diffused or sniffed, it is thought to reduce anxiety and depression. Many people incorporate this lovely scent into Reiki sessions to assist with immediate physical ailments, such as coughs, colds, flu, asthma, bronchitis, or sinus infections.

While diffusing essential oils during a Reiki session is recommended, be mindful of your clients and understand that essential oils do have side effects. Research the oils to learn which ones to avoid for certain medical conditions. For example, people with epilepsy or a risk of seizures should stay away from stimulating essential oils. Basil, cedarwood, cinnamon, fennel, and clove are stimulating essential oils you should avoid using during pregnancy.

YOGA

Yoga and Reiki pair very well together. Yoga, like Reiki, focuses on the natural flow of energy through the body. Many people first learn about the chakra system through yoga and are excited to further their understanding of energy work with Reiki.

Yoga teaches us all experiences reside in the chakras until they are healed. Unhealed physical, mental, and emotional traumas affect our physical health as well as our spiritual growth and can continue to grow and manifest into all sorts of ailments and disease.

Reiki can be used with yoga poses to send a concentrated boost of energy to selected chakras or power centers, increasing the flow of energy, boosting your practice, and breaking up blocks. Using Reiki to send energy through your body before, during, and after a yoga session will increase your flow of prana (life force energy) and accelerate the healing process.

So, just as specific yoga poses can unlock prana, rebalance the chakras, and bring about a spiritual awakening, including Reiki in your practice can dramatically increase your overall healing experience.

YIN YOGA

While Reiki pairs well with any type of yoga, I recommend you begin with Yin yoga. The term *Yin yoga* comes from the Taoist tradition of yin-yang balance. While yang relates to movement, creating heat in the body, yin is about finding stillness and cooling the body. Yin energy is something that we often need more of in our busy, stressed-out lives.

Yin yoga is accessible for all levels, and unlike Vinyasa and other popular yoga styles, in Yin all you need to do is relax in the pose. It is a soft, gentle way of giving up control, which is also something we learn from Reiki. We don't push or control the energy; we allow it to flow, just as in this type of yoga. Because this yoga style is slower and more relaxed, it allows you ample time to work with Reiki and really connect with the energy.

KUNDALINI YOGA

Kundalini yoga is more spiritual in nature. It is influenced by Shaktism and Tantra and is designed to help practitioners awaken their dormant Kundalini energy. This type of yoga incorporates chanting, meditation, breath work, mudras, and physical poses. *Kundalini* means "a spiritual energy or life force." This energy is thought to be located at the base of the spine and is frequently visualized as a coiled-up serpent, or snake.

Many people believe this is the same energy channeled via Reiki. The difference, of course, is this energy lies dormant within you, while Reiki pulls in life force energy from the cosmos.

Kundalini yoga moves the sleeping energy up from your base chakra through the crown chakra. Reiki can help the body prepare for this increase in power, as well as balance and refine the energy as it awakens and begins to rise. Working with Reiki will make the entire experience safer and more pleasurable.

PRANAYAMAS AND REIKI

Have you experienced pranayamas in your yoga practice? Pranayamas are specific breathing techniques and exercises used for balance, relaxation, and mental focus. We also use pranayama exercises to clear physical, mental, and emotional blocks in the body so that the breath and prana can flow freely. This controlled breath work also assists us in moving energy through the meridians (the energy pathways of the body) to the chakras.

When we include pranayamas in our Reiki practice, we create more life force energy and increase and refine our personal energy flow. This practice often works on our intuition because pranayamas work on the brain, too, balancing both the logical and creative hemispheres where our intuitive side lives. As we expand our abilities with Reiki, it is easier for us to step out of our own way. We stop micromanaging our experiences and second-guessing ourselves.

CHAKRA MEDITATION

Chakra meditations target specific chakras or all seven major chakras energy centers. These meditations can be done by visualizing the chakras, listening to a guided meditation, or chanting the seed syllable for the chakra. There are also chakra meditations that use a combination of all these techniques.

When we include Reiki in these meditations, we tap into the unlimited universal life force energy surrounding us. During meditation, we can direct this powerful energy to flow through the chakra system, removing blocks and realigning each center.

Reiki can empower your chakra meditation in new ways. Tapping into the Reiki energy during a chakra meditation often adds elements such as visions, sounds, or bodily sensations (such as tingles or shivers) as the energy moves through the body.

By committing to opening and balancing these energy centers, we are consciously working toward better health, as well as emotional and spiritual balance.

MEDITATION

A lot of people know the many benefits of meditation, yet so many people believe they don't have time to meditate. They feel they are too busy or have too much stress in their lives to even begin a meditation practice. But actually, the best time to meditate is when you feel stressed or over-whelmed. Reiki can help you relax into a meditation routine by facilitating a deep calm, allowing your body to unwind, making meditation much easier.

Combining Reiki and meditation also helps calm the mind. A clear, quiet, stress-free mind opens the door to going deeper into a state of inner peace and tranquility.

One easy way to complement your meditation practice is to sit in gassho (the Reiki meditation). Sit quietly, hands pressed together in front of your heart, silently repeating the Reiki precepts and allowing Reiki to run through your body. This meditation often ignites a flame of deep transformation and healing. We find our internal balance and are no longer worried, fearful, or consumed with negative thoughts or anger.

Meditation, especially coupled with Reiki, can help people cope with personal difficulties, overwhelming feelings, and stress. Reiki helps us reach a deeper state of physical and mental relaxation.

When adding Reiki to your meditation practice, you can find personal balance and feel less stressed or tense. Reiki assists us in reaching the calm and peaceful state that we are all searching for.

BREATH WORK

Breath work is a lovely and refreshing complement to your Reiki practice. While breath work and pranayama seem the same, there is a difference. Pranayama is breath work, but not all breath work is pranayama. By practicing pranayama, you control your breathing in order to achieve a certain state of meditation. In breath work, you can let your mind flow because you aren't after a meditative state. Breath work can also be done anywhere, at any time, to refresh and restore the physical body, and it boosts your spiritual senses.

Here is a simple but effective exercise you can try right now:

1. Begin by sitting up with your spine straight, either on the floor or in a chair with your feet in contact with the ground.

2. Check into Reiki and take a deep cleansing breath through the mouth. Release it through the nose. Repeat three times as you focus on your breath. (Never push or strain as you breathe.)

3. Now breathe normally and place your left hand lightly on your heart and your right hand softly on your lower belly.

4. Focus on your breath and allow your mind to clear as the Reiki flows.

5. Relax and focus on the rhythm of your breathing.

Breath work such as this calms the nervous system and soothes the body. Coupled with Reiki, simple breathing techniques can revitalize and energize your physical body.

WICCA AND WITCHCRAFT

Reiki can be paramount in opening up your personal consciousness and expanding your craft; Reiki and witchcraft both connect you to something bigger. With Reiki, we channel universal life force, which ties back to everything. This unlimited power source can be combined with witchcraft or other types of spell work.

I have taught and attuned many witches to Reiki to supplement their magical energy. They use Reiki for healing but also for consecrating herbal potions, charging candle spells, increasing protection charms, and for general spell work.

This powerful energy works well in tandem with rituals, goddess worship, ancestral magic, and other ceremonies. I often infuse my tarot cards with Reiki prior to a reading and use Reiki to cleanse space, enhance crystals, and energize food. Reiki can also empower objects, clear negativity, enhance intentions, and enchantments. It works well with nature and the planet, helping the environment return to a state of health and balance.

EVERYONE IS A TEACHER

The more we work with other people on their spiritual or healing path, the more we learn from their lives and personal experiences. Lessons are often related in the most unexpected places. As you tap into Reiki, you will soon attract more and more people into your life. Each client I have worked with has a unique perception of life, which can translate into powerful lessons on everything from everyday beliefs to huge spiritual truths.

Honor this gift by being fully present during a Reiki session. Listen without judgment and be open to the life lessons presented. Create a safe space for healing and growth. Know that the situation you are currently struggling with or the information you are looking for may be exactly what someone else is bringing into a session. Be open to learning from everyone.

The more you work with and practice Reiki, the more knowledge you acquire and the more you understand that everyone is a teacher. Read on to learn techniques for facilitating spiritual Reiki for yourself and others in the following chapters.

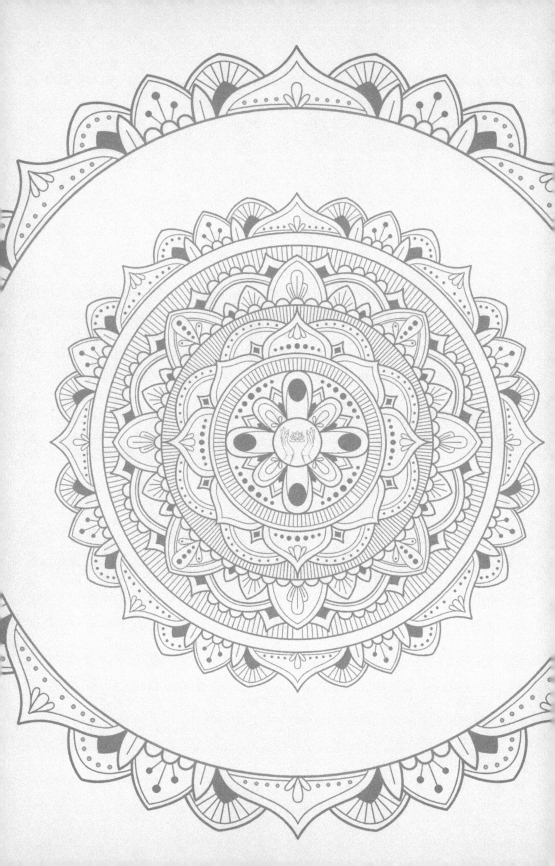

Part 2

Techniques for Spiritual Awakenings and Healing

Hand positions are fundamental in all schools of Reiki. Through specific hand positions, we send energy to targeted areas of the body. These positions assist in removing energy blocks, promoting wellness, easing pain, treating chronic conditions, and facilitating spiritual awakenings.

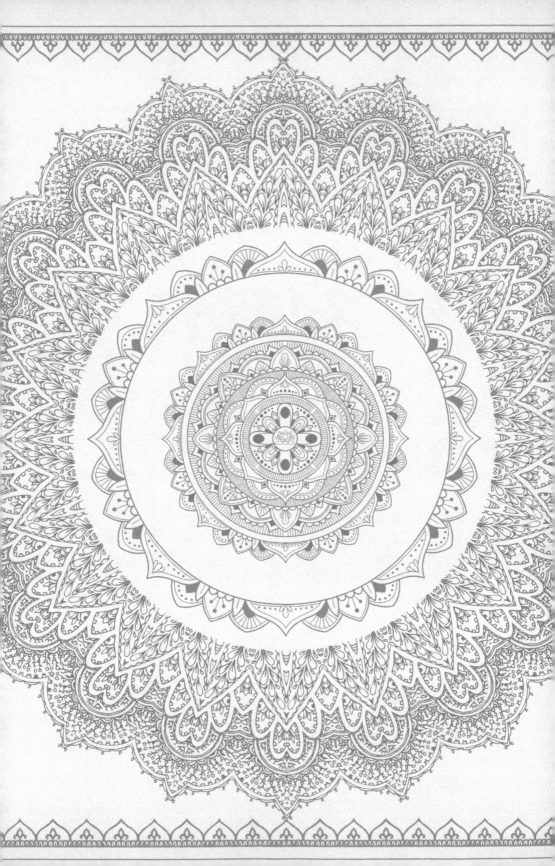

Chapter 6
Hand Positions for Self-Healing

I have included 15 hand positions that I use and teach in my Reiki level one class. These common hand positions make up one full Reiki session, but they are not mandatory or rigidly followed. They are meant to serve as a starting point for new Reiki students. These hand positions can be used any time to help refresh and restore the body. If you are feeling stressed or in pain, begin self-Reiki with these hand positions daily for optimum health, pain relief, and spiritual awakening.

Begin with these positions and stay in each one for about five minutes or longer as needed. Keep your mind clear and stay focused on sending Reiki.

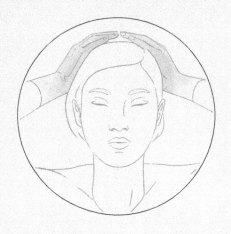

CROWN

Sitting up, place your hands on the top and along the sides of your head. Your fingers should be together, and you should cup your head comfortably with your hands. Your fingertips should just touch each other on the center of your head.

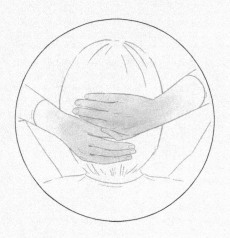

BACK OF HEAD

Stack your hands one above the other behind your head. Your bottom hand should be touching your neck, and your other hand should be just above it on the back of your skull.

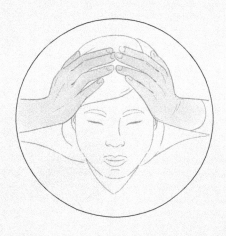

TEMPLES

Close your eyes and lightly place your hands on your temples. Your hands should be soft and your elbows relaxed.

EYES

Close your eyes and cup the hands lightly over the eyes. (Always avoid putting pressure on the tender eye area.) The palm chakra should be directly over each eye.

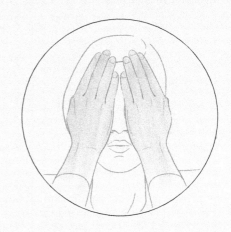

FACE

Using light touch and with your eyes closed, place your hands over your entire face. Keep your fingers together and resist the urge to apply pressure.

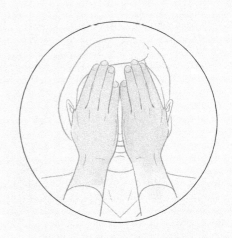

EARS

Place your hands on the sides of your face, covering your ears. Your fingers should be together and slightly cupped. Feeling pressure in your ears during this hand position is normal.

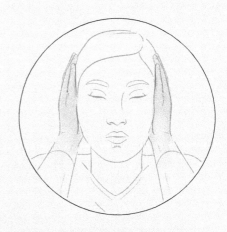

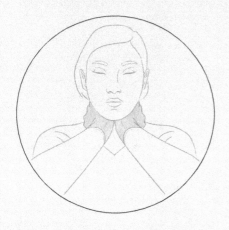

THROAT

While sitting up, gently rest your chin inside the palms of your cupped hands. Your hands should comfortably wrap along your jawline.

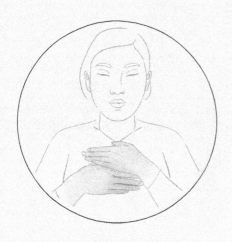

HEART

Place your left hand over your heart, extending slightly to the middle of your chest. Place your right hand slightly lower.

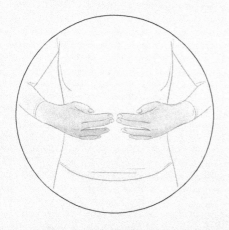

RIB CAGE

Sitting or lying on your back, place your cupped hands on your upper rib cage directly below your breasts. Relax your bent elbows.

SOLAR PLEXUS

Place your left hand comfortably in the middle of your body, just below your rib cage, with your right hand slightly below.

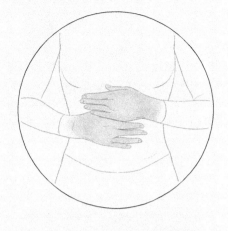

NAVEL

Place your left hand comfortably over your navel area, covering your belly button. Place your right hand right below your left hand.

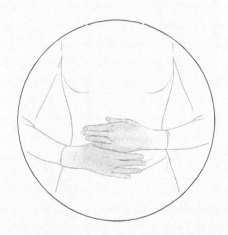

MID-BACK

Standing up, reach behind your back with elbows bent and place your hands on the center of your back.

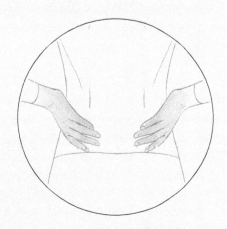

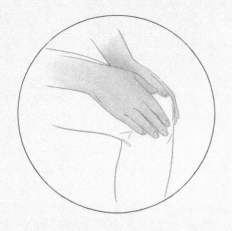

KNEES

Sitting comfortably, cup each hand around your left knee. After 5 to 10 minutes move your hands to your right knee, repeating the same hand position.

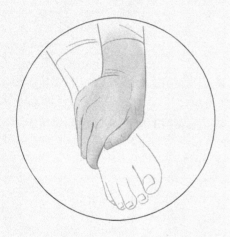

ANKLES

Place your left hand gently on your ankle. Repeat after 5 to 10 minutes with your right hand on your right ankle.

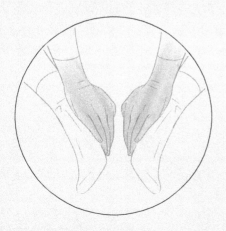

SOLES OF THE FEET

Sitting comfortably, place your hands on the soles of each foot. Gently grip each foot and allow the Reiki to flow.

While this might seem like a lot for a personal Reiki session, remember a little Reiki is better than no Reiki. If, for example, you are stuck in traffic, you can easily Reiki your crown, ears, or throat while sitting in your car.

Ideally, we should make time each day to complete a full self-Reiki session, but if that is impossible, any amount of Reiki will be helpful.

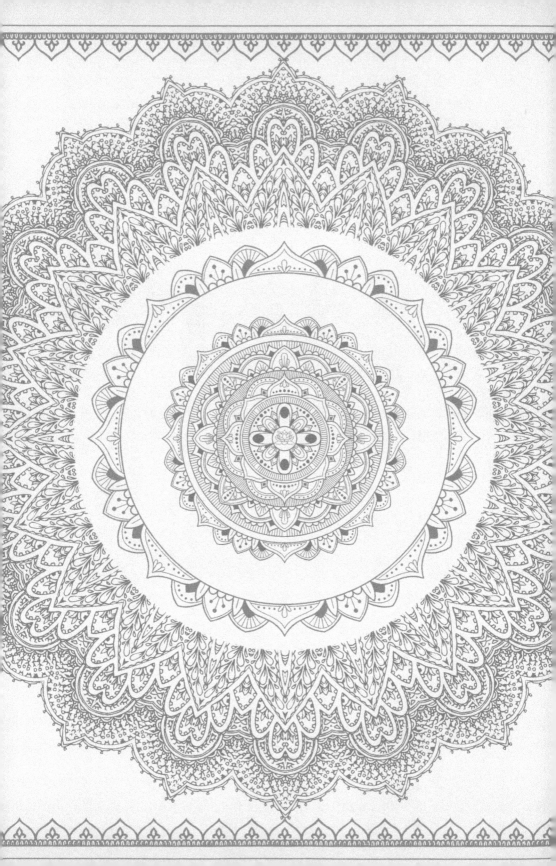

Chapter 7
Hand Positions for Healing Others

In this chapter, you will find hand positions for healing others. This system of hand sequences is based on current Reiki hand positions used in the West. Combining what I learned in Reiki classes with personal experience in treating thousands of people, these positions have become my go-to sequences for treating others. These positions are effective for treating most common ailments, reducing pain levels, and addressing mental/emotional issues. They can be used in a full-body session or as spot treatments on the fly.

When practicing on others, make sure your clients are comfortable and able to relax during the session. Some people prefer quiet, while others like to talk during a session. Follow your instincts with each client. Also allow them ample space to ask questions or express what they are feeling. As a practitioner, make sure you stay positive and grounded in the moment. (No drifting off thinking about your problems or to-do list.)

This intelligent energy will go where it is most needed and do the most good. Remember, you cannot get too much Reiki, so when in doubt, stay longer over the affected area of the body. Let's Reiki!

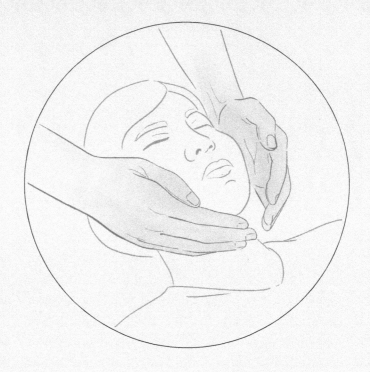

HEAD

This position is the starting position unless the client has diabetes; in that case, we begin with the feet. It is useful in treating headaches, stress, worry, and an overactive mind. Become quiet and connect with Reiki. If possible, the client should be lying face up on a massage table or sitting up comfortably. Place your hands on or hover around the side of the head, keeping your fingers together. Your palm chakra should be around the ear area and your hands should lightly hover about one inch from the client's head. Allow the energy to flow from your palm chakras and fingertips. Always keep your mind as clear as possible when working on someone's head.

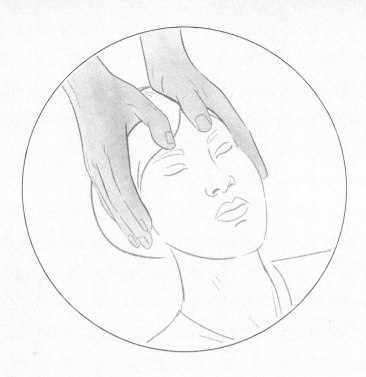

CROWN

This position is useful for treating migraine pain, sadness, stress, and burnout. From the starting position, standing behind the client, move your hands back toward your own body and the client's crown, or the top of the head. Your thumbs would then be just above the client's eyebrow area. If using full touch, be very gentle.

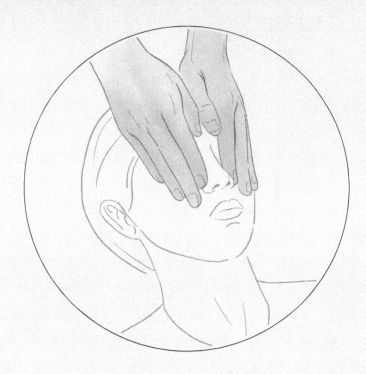

FACE

This position is useful in treating sinus pain, toothache, vision problems, and Bell's palsy. Keeping your fingers together, cover the client's face lightly with your hands. Do not put pressure on the face. Your palm chakra should be directly over the eyes. It is common for folks to see flashes of light, colors, or images when you are over the face. Let clients know this is a safe space and they are free to discuss what they are seeing.

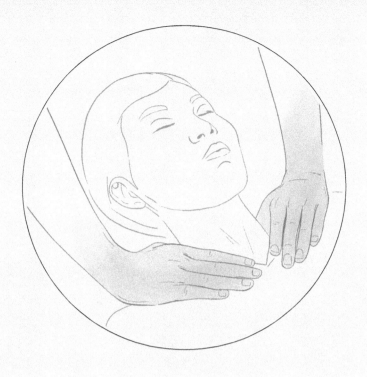

TOP OF THE SHOULDER

This position is useful for treating back pain, muscle tension, insomnia, and stress. Using light touch, place your hand on the client's collarbone. Your fingers should come together just below the hollow of the throat. You may feel the client's body relax at this point. We often walk around carrying the weight of the world on our shoulders. Sending energy to this part of the body can make a huge difference in stress levels.

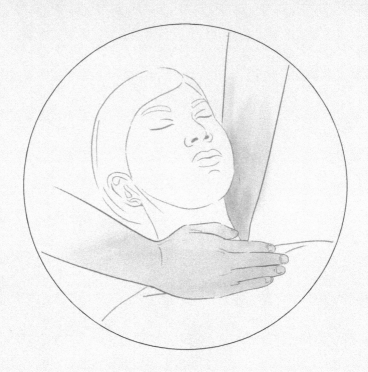

THROAT

This position is useful for treating acid reflux, sore throat, heartburn, speech and anxiety issues, and fear of public speaking. We also work with this chakra to help clients feel more empowered and heard in their relationships. Gently place your hand above the hollow of the throat with the other hand on the back of the neck. (It doesn't matter which hand is placed where, as Reiki flows equally through either hand.) Remember, many people are uncomfortable having their throats touched, so be mindful of the client's comfort level in this delicate area.

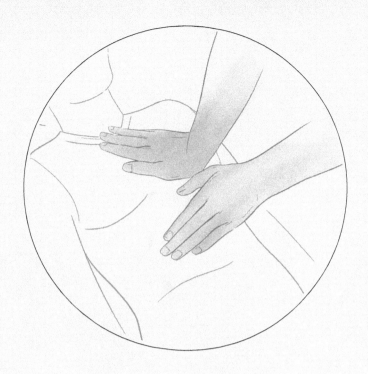

HEART

This position is useful for treating heart issues, emotional overload, relationship problems, and issues of self-confidence and self-worth. Remember, we never treat anyone with a pacemaker as the energy can interfere with the battery of the pacemaker. Place one hand flat, palm down, about two inches above the middle of the chest, being mindful of the client's comfort level. Place your other hand just under it and turned out slightly.

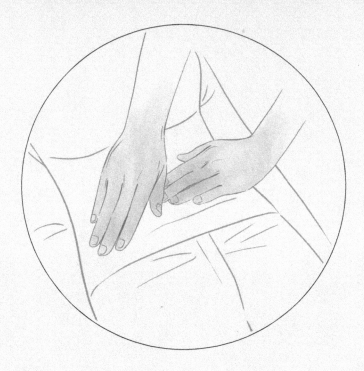

STOMACH

This position is useful for treating digestive issues, irritable bowel syndrome, fear, anxiety, and issues related to worry and dread. Place your hands lightly on the client's stomach. Your fingers should be together with hands facing in the same direction as you treat the stomach area.

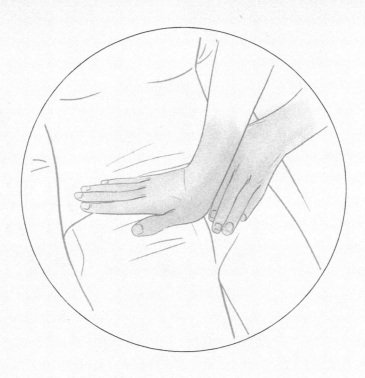

LOWER STOMACH

This position is useful for treating digestive issues, panic, fear, anger, incontinence, bladder issues, reproductive issues, and past-life issues. Hover your hands lightly over the area just under the belly button. Keep your fingers together and your hands slightly cupped. Be mindful of your client's comfort level. When in doubt, choose modesty.

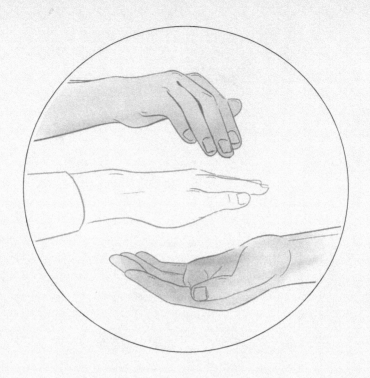

HANDS

This position is useful in treating carpal tunnel syndrome, arthritic joints, fear, sensitivity, headaches, chronic pain, and sadness. Hover slightly above the client's left hand with your hands sandwiching the client's outstretched hand. Repeat with the right hand in the same manner.

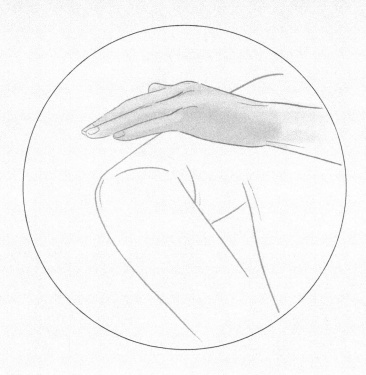

ELBOWS

Place one hand above the client's elbow and one underneath it. Allow the joint to take as much energy as needed. Issues with the elbow could represent the ability to change direction in our life, so don't skip this one! Repeat on the other elbow, staying in this position as long as needed.

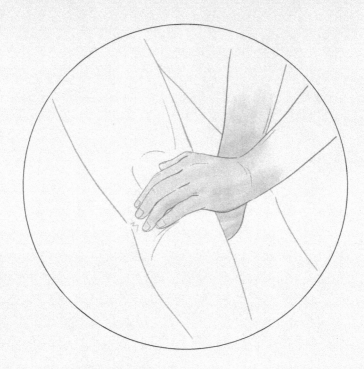

KNEES

This position is used for knee injuries and energy blockage in the lower body and for when a person feels stuck in life. Begin by placing one hand on the kneecap and the other, if possible, under the knee. Work on one leg, and when the energy is balanced, move to the opposite leg.

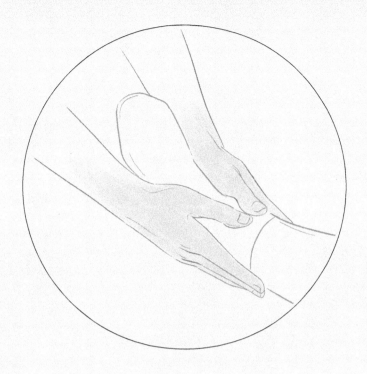

ANKLES

This position is useful for treating joint issues, fear, emotional issues, personal development, and grief. Place both hands lightly around the left ankle, then the right one. Note that when you're in this position, clients will likely draw energy from your lower three chakras and your hands from the bottom of their feet. Clients are unaware their bodies are doing this, and it is completely involuntary. It will not harm you; just make sure you are fully grounded and using Reiki.

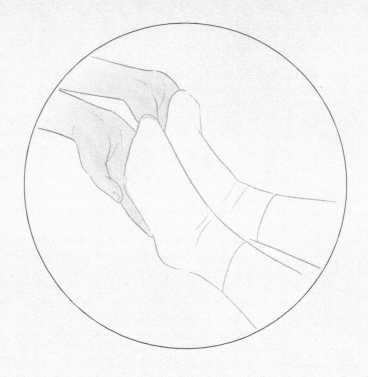

FEET

This position helps re-energize a fatigued person and aids in grounding, uncovering emotional blocks, and restoring failing health. Begin by checking into Reiki and have the client remove their shoes (socks are fine). Move to Reiki the bottom of each foot, paying special attention to the large chakra in the middle of the foot. If you cannot feel a pull or draw from this chakra, place the power symbol on the chakra (beginning with the right foot) and with two fingers, make clockwise turns, as if you were screwing in a corkscrew. Mentally count to nine. On the ninth round, unscrew the symbol, repeating the motion counterclockwise. Next, send Reiki to the chakra again for five to seven minutes. This may cause the foot chakra to drain. It may feel as if the energy is suddenly flowing out of the foot like an open tap. This opening is not draining the client's energy; it is allowing old, stuck energy to be released.

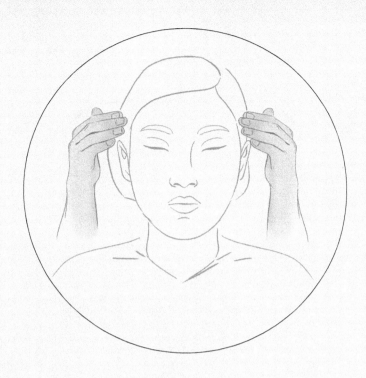

FOR GENERAL WELL-BEING

Once you are centered, grounded, and calm, draw the power symbol over the middle of the body with your finger. From there, stand behind the client and place both hands beside the client's temples, one hand on each side, about two inches away from the head. It is very important to keep your mind blank when you are working on someone's head. If your mind wanders, mentally repeat *Reiki* over and over until your mind settles. Stay in this position for at least seven minutes, although you can stay longer. Move your hands to cover the client's ears. Finally, hover over the back of the skull. (You can also touch the ears or the back of the skull if your client consents to that.)

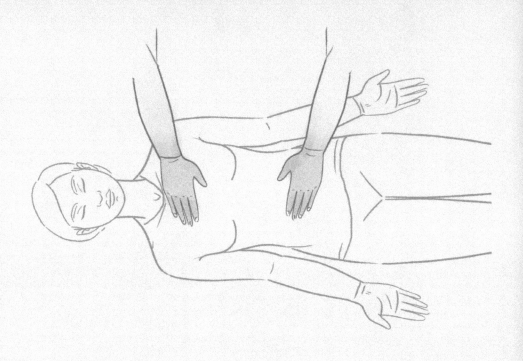

SMOOTH THE CLIENT'S AURA

This is usually done after each full Reiki session. Upon completing a full session, gently sweep your client's aura with your hands by moving your hands about three to four inches over the body. If the client is restless and anxious, we sweep away from the hara line. If the client is listless, overwhelmed, or exhausted, we sweep toward the middle of the body. Next, we pack the energy down lightly with the palms and then smooth it.

Be sure to tell your clients to drink more water for 24 hours after the session. The Reiki should continue to work on their energy for five to seven days after the actual energy session ends. Most often clients feel very relaxed and experience a more restful, restorative sleep and a deep sense of peace and acceptance.

Occasionally, an energy session may bring up trauma or past pain that is ready to be released. When this happens, the client may experience a healing crisis and a powerful cleansing afterward. Make sure your client knows this experience is normal and that you are available.

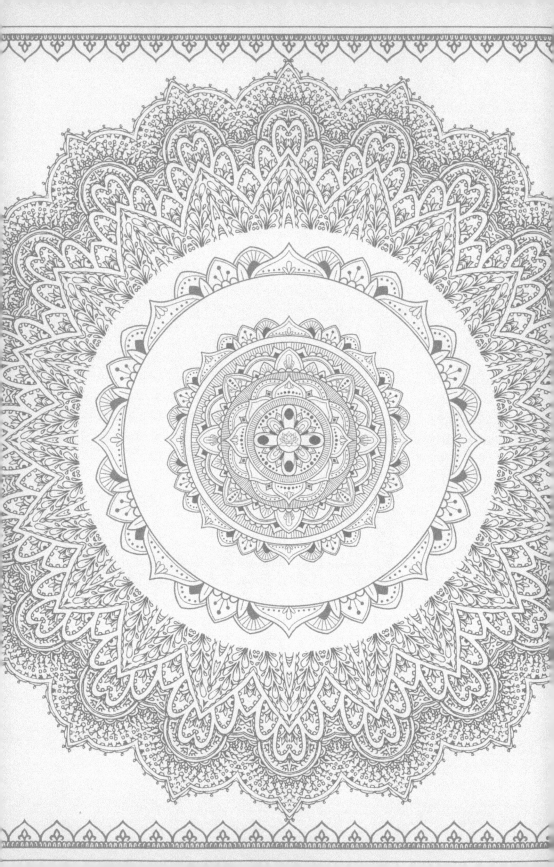

Chapter 8

Sequences for Enhancing and Awakening Spiritual Experiences

In this chapter, you will find Reiki hand positions for enhancing and awakening spiritual experiences. You may use these hand positions with clients or for self-Reiki. Begin with chakra balancing, then move on to more targeted techniques, such as the sequences for building your intuitive muscles, for ascension symptoms, or for opening the way for personal evolution.

Remember to go through the sequences slowly and thoughtfully. As in yoga, never push or strain. Be patient and listen to your body. As you move from one sequence to the next, slide your hands from one position to another as smoothly as you can and keep your mind clear.

Allow yourself time to become accustomed to the personal energy changes Reiki will bring into your life and remember spiritual awakening comes on its own timetable. As you work toward balancing your energy, you can expect all levels of your life to change and improve.

ROOT CHAKRA SUPPORT

The root chakra is key to understanding our physical place in the world, our fight-or-flight response, and our connection to our ancestors. It is often overlooked in favor of working on the higher chakras, but to facilitate spiritual experiences, this chakra must be in balance. Take the time to balance and heal this chakra to ensure energy can flow to the higher chakras and address your physical needs.

1 Connect with Reiki and place your hands at the base of your spine or tailbone.

2 Close your eyes and imagine red light coming down from heaven, flooding this chakra with healing energy. Hold this position for 10 to 15 minutes or longer.

SACRAL CHAKRA SUPPORT

Sending Reiki to this chakra can shift how we perceive ourselves and begin a healthy flow of self-acceptance and empowerment. Nurture yourself as you would a dear friend.

1 Connect to Reiki and place your hands side by side over the lower abdomen, a few inches below the navel.

2 Stay in this position for at least 10 minutes with your eyes closed, allowing the energy to flow. Don't judge or discount any images or sensations that come up during this position.

SOLAR PLEXUS CHAKRA SUPPORT

Sending Reiki to this chakra helps us deal with raw, unsettled, or unaddressed emotions such as frustration, anger, and rage. It is possible that you may understand the cause or reason for these feelings and new ways of dealing with situations after balancing this energy center.

❶ Place hands side by side just above the navel and allow the Reiki to flow. You may notice heat flowing from your hands at this chakra because it is often underactive in people. (If you don't feel this, it's okay. That doesn't mean the Reiki isn't working; we all experience things differently.)

❷ Hold this position for 10 to 15 minutes or as needed.

HEART CHAKRA SUPPORT

The heart chakra can be another area where we hold fear, shock, or trauma, and these issues may come up after a treatment. Allow the experience to unfold without judgment. If you feel like crying, cry. If you feel like laughing, laugh.

Trust the process and allow yourself, as you would a loved one, the time and space you require to process heart issues. Know that you are loved and that you matter.

❶ Place a piece of tumbled turquoise or a piece of jewelry in the center of your chest.

❷ Place your hands side by side about one to two inches above the upper heart area. Close your eyes and allow the energy to flow. Stay in this position for at least 10 minutes with your eyes closed. Don't judge or discount any images or sensations that come up during this position.

THROAT CHAKRA SUPPORT

This delicate chakra is often blocked in men and almost always blocked in women. The throat chakra is key to stepping into your power and embracing your abilities. Signs this chakra is opening during a Reiki session include coughing, sneezing, hiccupping, choking on words, or laughing. All are natural reactions to the energy flowing freely through the chakra.

❶ Gently place one hand above the hollow of the throat and the other hand on the back of the neck. Lightly grip your throat with the palm chakra facing your throat chakra. Stay in this position as long as it is comfortable.

❷ As an alternative, you may place your other hand over the heart instead of the back of the neck. This could be an uncomfortable position, and you may not be able to hold it long, which is fine. Stay in it only as long as you feel comfortable.

THIRD EYE CHAKRA SUPPORT

This is a powerful position for opening your spiritual abilities. This position also stimulates the face, nose, eyes, sinuses, and lymphatic system and is useful for stress, burnout, and hormone imbalances. It opens up intuitive abilities and creativity. Signs this chakra is opening during a Reiki session include a light tickle or itch in the middle of the forehead, seeing flashes of light, seeing shadows out of the

❶ Get comfortable and close your eyes.

❷ Connect to Reiki and place both hands gently over your eyes. Remember to not use any pressure over the eyes. Hold this position for 10 to 15 minutes or for as long as needed.

corner of the eye, and a wider field of peripheral vision. Your eyesight may also improve, and colors may look much more intense and vibrant.

CROWN CHAKRA SUPPORT

The crown chakra is associated with the brain, including the pituitary gland, the pineal gland, and the hypothalamus, as well as the nervous system. Sending energy to this chakra further connects us to our community, intuition, guides, and divine wisdom. When this chakra is in balance, we can easily tap into higher consciousness, wisdom, and the divine. But for enough energy to pass through the higher

1 Check into Reiki and place your hands on each side of your head. Your palms should be over your temples. Be careful not to apply any pressure.

2 Hold this position for at least 10 minutes.

CONTINUED

chakras, we cannot neglect the lower energy centers. It is important to include all seven major chakras in a full energy session whenever possible.

CHAKRA CLEARING ENERGY PATHWAYS

Use this hand position for balancing and easing blockages that are slowing or stopping the flow of energy through the chakras.

1 If possible, lie facedown on a massage table and relax.

2 Connect with Reiki and place one hand at the base of the neck and the other on the small of the back. Send Reiki and visualize the energy flowing from your root chakra to the crown and back again. See the energy remove all blocks as it becomes more refined as it passes through each chakra. Hold the position for 10 to 15 minutes or for as long as it is comfortable. You should feel Reiki energizing and rebalancing each energy center as it clears the energy pathway.

FOR SPIRITUAL AWAKENING

This sequence may open your third eye, and you may see colors, visions, or images. Journal your experience and note any synchronicity that follows this session, such as seeing repeating numbers, sensing someone is about to text, or feeling the emotions of others. Practice this sequence along with a full-body Reiki session weekly to increase and open yourself up to more spiritual encounters and experiences.

1 Lie on your back in a comfortable position. You may bend your knees or use a pillow for your head.

2 Place a small piece of Reiki-infused clear quartz in the center of your chest (a pendant or a small piece of raw quartz works well).

3 Check into Reiki, cup your hands and place a hand on each side of your head. Use gentle pressure and close your eyes.

4 In your mind's eye, see the power symbol hovering above and in front of you. Allow the energy of the power symbol to float or move. It may land on your body or on a chakra point. It may take practice to see it. The more you meditate, the easier seeing the symbol will be. Hold this position for 10 to 20 minutes or as needed.

FOR RESTORING THE BODY AFTER A SPIRITUAL EXPERIENCE

It is important to take care of yourself when you are experiencing spiritual encounters or your abilities are developing. One simple way to do this is to incorporate crystals into your self-Reiki routine.

1 Have the client hold a Reiki-programmed rose quartz stone in each hand. If you're doing self-Reiki, lay the stones on your lap.

2 From a sitting position, begin Reiking the feet for five to seven minutes. If possible, bend your leg and place both hands on your foot, sending Reiki to the top and instep of the foot. If this isn't a comfortable position, you may just send Reiki to the bottom of the foot.

3 Once you have sent energy to both feet, draw the power symbol in the air over the top of the left foot.

4 Reiki the top of the foot. Stay in this position as long as needed, noticing how the body takes the energy.

5 Move your hand to the ankle and send Reiki for another five to seven minutes.

6 Repeat the procedure on the right foot.

7 Move your hands to the tailbone and send Reiki. Continue to send energy for five to seven minutes or as needed.

8 End the session by drinking water and continue to increase your water intake throughout the day.

⑨ Journal your experiences and repeat this sequence daily until your energy is rebalanced and you feel stronger. Don't push yourself or try to do too much spiritually. It takes time to integrate new energy and abilities.

FOR MANIFESTING A POSITIVE OUTCOME

If you are stressed or worried over a problem, practice this hand sequence.

❶ Check into Reiki and place your hands on your shoulders.
❷ Close your eyes. In your mind's eye, see the positive outcome you wish to obtain, such as a bid on a new house being accepted, a medical test showing a positive outcome, or a new automobile.
❸ Next, place your hands on the hara chakra (on the front of the body) and allow the Reiki to flow. After about 10 minutes, move your hands to the back and Reiki the hara chakra from this position.
❹ When finished, drink a glass of water and let go of all fear and worry surrounding the situation.

TO MOVE FORWARD

If you are feeling stuck or unsure of your life's direction, go through this sequence. After this session, most people notice an almost immediate shift; they feel more empowered and find it easier to move forward.

❶ Remove your shoes and check into Reiki.

❷ Close your eyes and visualize yourself moving forward. See yourself doing new things and having new, exciting adventures. You are successful and powerful.

❸ In your mind's eye, see the long-distance symbol and the power symbol floating over you.

❹ Open your eyes and bend over like you are tying your shoes. Trace the power symbol over the top of each foot and lightly blow it into place. Exhale slowly like you are blowing out a candle and see the symbol float to the top of each foot.

❺ Reiki your feet for 10 to 15 minutes daily until you feel you are moving forward and notice positive changes in your life.

FOR BUILDING YOUR INTUITIVE MUSCLES—SEEING

This sequence may work almost instantly, allowing you to see more colors, shapes, and images out of the corner of your eye. You may also notice that your dreams are more vivid and intense and that you have more control over them. It is likely that your dreams will become more like full-length films and include deeper, magical themes. Often as we begin to see, our dreams become less rooted in our subconscious and more intense. You may also notice an improvement in eyesight and your field of vision.

1   Connect with Reiki and state your intention to the Universe, such as *I clearly see myself and everything around me.*

2   Place your hands over your eyes with your thumbs together over the bridge of the nose. Hold for at least five to seven minutes.

3   Move your dominant hand to back of the neck and continue to Reiki the third eye chakra. Stay in this position for as long as you're comfortable.

4   Do not repeat this sequence more than once per week as it takes time to adjust to seeing. If you become alarmed or frightened by what you are seeing, skip a month and allow your body and mind time to process this new information. Don't rush the process.

FOR BUILDING YOUR INTUITIVE ABILITIES—FEELING

This sequence will open up your senses and allow more information to pass through the lower chakras. As the chakras move back into alignment, you should experience more and more moments of being in the flow—moments when you feel events, people, places, and things around you in a deeper and more meaningful way. You will understand things from a spiritual viewpoint, not just a physical or logical sense. When we tap into our intuitive senses, we feel connected to something bigger.

❶ Stand up and check into Reiki.

❷ Send Reiki to the upper spine by placing your hands behind the back. Hold for five minutes.

❸ Move your hands to the mid-back. Hold for five to seven minutes.

❹ Move your hands to the lower waist. Hold for as long as it's comfortable.

❺ Journal your experiences.

❻ Note all changes, even small things like being able to pick up on your friends' emotions, finding a great parking space, or sensing changes in the weather, as these are probably signs of more abilities that will soon be opening up for you. Besides improving your ability to feel energy around you, this sequence will alleviate isolation and loneliness issues. You will become more attuned to the divine energy that flows through everything.

CONNECT TO
ANGELIC BEINGS

You can deepen your connection to or form a bond with angelic beings using Reiki. Remember, angelic beings, guides, and ancestors will never tell you to harm yourself or anyone else—when in doubt, use discernment. This energy can be powerful and should not be overused. Do this session no more than once per week.

❶ Ground and connect to Reiki.

❷ Find a comfortable place to sit where you will not be disturbed for 15 to 20 minutes.

❸ Place Reiki-infused pieces of amber, golden topaz, and clear quartz around you. (Use one of each crystal.)

❹ Set a timer for 20 minutes and move into a meditative state.

❺ With your eyes closed, see in your mind's eye a spotlight of golden light pour down from the sky. When you see the light, call on the archangel Michael or any angelic beings you wish to connect with.

❻ Sit quietly and allow the energy to engulf you. Be open to the energy and do not judge it. Allow the experience to unfold in its own way without expectation.

❼ When the timer goes off, end the session by saying thank you for the experience and see the light travel back up into the sky, breaking the connection.

❽ Journal any messages or visions you may have received.

FOR BALANCING PERSONAL ENERGY

Use this sequence when you feel scattered, off balance, overly emotional, or fatigued. Easy-to-find stones that can help dissolve blockages and amplify healing energy are quartz, amethyst, citrine, purple fluorite, and carnelian. These can be worn as jewelry or held during meditation and energy healing. This sequence also makes a wonderful weekly self-care routine to help combat feeling stressed and overwhelmed.

1 Give yourself 20 to 30 minutes of quiet in a calm place where you will not be disturbed.

2 Shut off all electronics and check into Reiki.

3 Take a deep breath and release it slowly, sending energy to your left elbow. After five minutes, switch to the right elbow.

4 Move your hands to Reiki the tops of your shoulders. Relax and allow the energy to flow for an additional 7 to 10 minutes.

5 Move your hands to Reiki your feet. Your mind should be calm by this point, and you should feel an overall physical energy shift. Take your time and send energy to your feet for as long as needed.

6 Sit for a few minutes and just allow the energy to flow. You should feel a mood shift or a change in your emotions when the energy shifts. Do not be in a hurry to go back to your day. Allow yourself time to recover.

FOR ASCENSION SYMPTOMS

Ascension symptoms can show up as flu-like symptoms that come and go, headaches, muscle pains, and general fatigue. A full, hour-long session is recommended for ascension symptoms, but if you do not have the time, try this simple sequence. If the symptoms persist, seek medical care.

❶ Find a quiet place, preferably a dark room, turn off all electronics, and loosen any tight or restrictive clothing.

❷ Connect to Reiki and Reiki the root chakra for at least 10 minutes.

❸ Move to the heart chakra with one hand on the throat chakra. Stay in this position for five to seven minutes. Remember that in Reiki we never cross our hands or legs. We always keep everything soft but in alignment so the energy can flow freely.

❹ Finish this session off by Reiking the third eye chakra. Send energy for 7 to 10 minutes or for as long as needed.

❺ Drink a bottle of pure water after the session and give yourself time to rest. Stay away from processed food and stressful situations.

❻ Reiki should not replace medical care but complement it. If you are still feeling ill, seek medical treatment.

FOR MENTAL/EMOTIONAL ASCENSION SYMPTOMS

If your symptoms are more emotional in nature and you have stressful, worried thoughts for no apparent reason, flashbacks of past traumas, and over-the-top fatigue, try this sequence.

1 Take three deep breaths in through the nose. Gently exhale through the mouth like you are blowing out a candle.

2 Breathe normally and lie down comfortably in a dark room where you will be alone and can be in a quiet place for the length of the session.

3 Connect to Reiki and send energy to your elbows for 10 to 15 minutes each. Allow the energy to flow. Don't try to suppress your thoughts; instead, gently push them away, not letting them hook your attention.

4 Move to Reiki your shoulders. Stay in this position for 10 minutes or longer.

5 Finish off by moving to Reiki the hara chakra. Stay in this position for 10 to 15 minutes or longer if needed.

6 When your mind becomes peaceful, sit in gassho and repeat the Reiki precepts.

7 Remember to drink more water when you are going through ascension and make time to rest.

TO ACCESS PAST-LIFE MEMORIES

For this sequence, you will need a piece of amethyst, a recorder or an app that will record your session, and about 25 minutes alone in a calm and quiet area. Because this sequence can be rather intense, limit it to only once per week. It is best to schedule it on the weekend or a quiet day, as you will need time to rest afterward.

1 Connect to Reiki and state your intention, something like *I wish to connect with my past-life memories in a way that I can understand and easily remember.*

2 Lie comfortably on your back and set a timer for 25 minutes.

3 Record the session and speak out loud. Verbalize any impressions, sensations, information, or emotions that come up.

4 Place a piece of Reiki-infused amethyst in the center of your forehead.

5 Close your eyes and quiet your mind.

6 Send Reiki to the sides of your head for five to seven minutes.

7 Move your hands and begin hovering over your third eye chakra for another 10 to 15 minutes.

8 Rest your arms comfortably at your sides and allow your breathing to soften. Be open to seeing colors, images, and places. Describe what you see out loud for the recording.

9 End the session when the timer goes off and drink a glass of water. Review the recording and journal your memories.

POST–TRAUMATIC STRESS DISORDER

Reiki can be used along with cognitive therapy, shadow work, or other types of therapy.

❶ Begin by going through the full body session described in chapter 7. Spend as long as needed in each position.

❷ Repeat the entire session every three days for at least a month.

❸ Make time to meditate on the Reiki precepts daily.

❹ Begin writing down your thoughts, memories, and emotions every day.

❺ Reiki isn't intended to replace proper medical care, but it works in tandem with it to accelerate self-healing. Listen to your body and seek appropriate care when needed.

BEFORE A TAROT READING

Reiki can support you in giving a better card reading!

❶ Before you begin a card reading, ground yourself and check into Reiki.

❷ Place your hand over the entire deck and send Reiki to it.

❸ State the intention that the reading will be truthful, helpful, and guided by Spirit.

❹ Drink a few sips of water and begin the session.

❺ Repeat before each reading.

BEFORE CRAFT/ SPELL WORK

Reiki can empower and enhance craft work and assist you in staying present and focused.

1. Find a quiet place and ground yourself to the earth. Imagine that you have tree roots coming out of the bottoms of your feet and tailbone; they are going miles down into the earth to connect with the core of the planet.

2. Say to yourself *I am grounded and present in my body*. You should instantly feel more clearheaded and focused.

3. Check into Reiki.

4. Lightly place one hand over the throat chakra and your other hand over your heart for about 10 minutes.

5. Reiki each of your hands.

6. Set the intention that your craft or spell work will be infused with the highest energy, harming none.

BEFORE CHANNELING

Reiki can help you calm your mind and strengthen your ability to channel. It's important to take care of yourself when doing vibrational energy work. Always allow yourself time to rest between sessions and know your limits.

1. Find a quiet, out-of-the-way place and ground yourself.
2. Check into Reiki and send the energy to the bottoms of your feet for seven to nine minutes.
3. Move to your heart chakra position, staying over this energy center for five to seven minutes.
4. Place one palm on your forehead and the other on the back of your head. Spend five to seven minutes, or longer, in this position.
5. Set the intention that you will be a safe and secure channel for truthful information.
6. When your channeling session is over, make sure you break the energetic connection and drink plenty of water.
7. Give yourself time to rest and recover in between sessions.

FOR SELF-AWARENESS

There are times when we need answers and they just won't come forward. For example, if you are unsure of a job offer, a proposal, or even what vitamins you should be taking, self-awareness could help. Try this exercise to tap into your body's inner wisdom and awareness.

1 Ground and check into Reiki.

2 Take a series of deep breaths and then breathe normally.

3 Sit comfortably on the floor if possible. If not, sit with bare feet touching the floor.

4 Place your hands in front of your chest as if in prayer. Clear your mind and relax.

5 Repeat the Reiki precepts slowly and with conviction.

6 Next, place one hand on your heart and one hand on your forehead for about six minutes. Open your mind to receiving information in whatever form it takes. Do not judge any information that comes to you; just note it. (It may show up as memories, written words, remembered conversations, television programs, or songs.)

7 After the session has ended, journal any messages, images, or visions you saw and drink a glass of pure water.

FOR MANIFESTING

Reiki can empower your manifesting and help you manifest the life you dream of!

① Take a few deep breaths and ground yourself to the earth.

② Clear your mind and check into Reiki.

③ Place a piece of Reiki-infused malachite over your heart. (A pendant works well, but it can also be a tumbled piece you carry in your shirt or bra.)

④ Place your hands on your shoulders, but do not cross your arms. Send Reiki for 15 minutes.

⑤ Move to your heart chakra, continuing to send energy for at least seven minutes.

⑥ Finish with five to seven minutes of Reiki to the crown chakra.

⑦ As you finish the session, think or say out loud, *I accept abundance and prosperity into my life.*

⑧ After the session, take a small, clean piece of paper and write what it is specifically you want to manifest, such as a new car, a vacation, or a better job. For instance, if you want to go on vacation, write down where you want to go and how long you will be there. *I want to take a vacation in April in Sedona. My family will stay one week and have a wonderful time.*

9 Send Reiki to the paper and draw the power symbol on the back, then fold the paper nine times and carry it with you in your wallet or purse.

10 Wear or carry the malachite with you and sleep with it under your pillow or on your nightstand.

11 Repeat daily until you have manifested your goal.

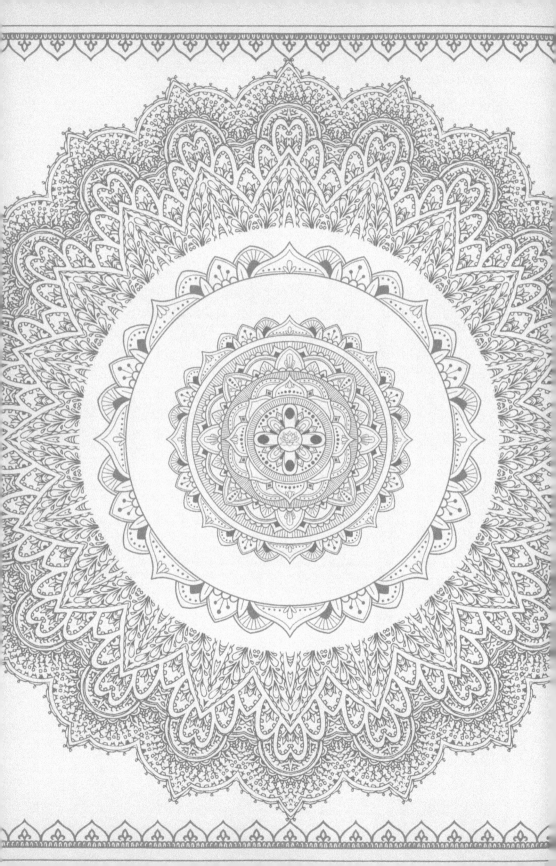

Chapter 9

Sequences for Spiritual and Emotional Healing

In this chapter, we will review some simple and effective ways to use Reiki for spiritual empowerment and mental and emotional healing. Many of these sequences require multiple hand positions and other complementary additions like breath work, crystals, and affirmations.

We often look at mental health as a stigma, but I believe we need to focus on mental wellness. We are emotional animals by nature. We have all come here to learn and evolve, which requires that we have emotions and emotional experiences. I have included some simple hand positions as well as meditations and exercises to help you engage with Reiki as you understand and heal some of these issues. As always, Reiki should not replace medical care but should be used as a complement to it. If you are having suicidal thoughts or suffering from lingering depression, please seek medical help. We want you healthy and strong.

FOR SHIELDING

Reiki can be used as a shield to stop unwanted energy from attaching to you. Repeat this sequence daily.

❶ Stand up, raise your arms over your head, and connect to Reiki.

❷ Close your eyes and imagine a large, translucent ray of light pouring down from heaven onto you. See it in your mind's eye as the embodiment of Reiki flooding down around you.

❸ Call on your guides, angels, source, or higher self to connect with the Reiki and shield you throughout the day. Allow this powerful energy to totally engulf you.

TO RELEASE ANXIETY

Reiki can be used to help anxiety and anxiety attacks. If you are currently taking medication, please continue to take your prescribed dosage. If you feel the Reiki is lessening the anxiety and you may no longer need the medication, inform your doctor before altering your dosage.

❶ Drink a class of pure water, then connect with Reiki.

❷ Place one hand on your brow, lightly covering the third eye, and one hand in the middle of your chest, covering the heart chakra. Send energy for about 10 minutes.

❸ Move both hands to your upper chest, slightly above the heart chakra. Breathe deeply and calmly as you continue to Reiki this area. Repeat the affirmation *I live a calm, peaceful life.*

❹ Repeat this sequence before stressful events or as needed.

GRIEF

Reiki can help lessen the effects of grief. If you are currently grieving, Reiki will not take the pain away but it can help you manage it. Remember, grief is a process, and there will be good days and bad days as you move through it. Use this sequence for emotional support as needed.

❶ Find a quiet place where you will not be disturbed and check into Reiki.

❷ Put on some soothing instrumental music and repeat the affirmation *I accept my life and allow the feeling of peace to wash over me.*

❸ Begin the Reiki session by placing your hands on the heart chakra. Spend at least 7 to 10 minutes in this position.

❹ Reiki the throat for an additional 7 to 10 minutes.

❺ Move to the crown and Reiki for at least 7 to 10 minutes or for as long as you feel comfortable.

❻ If you feel emotional, allow the emotions to come to the surface. Cry, yell, scream, or whatever else you feel you need to do. Bottling the emotions up or trying to suppress them will do more harm than good.

❼ After the session is over, journal your feelings from a place of nonjudgment. You are allowed to feel the way you do. By doing regular Reiki sessions, you will slowly come back into balance and find peace.

STRESS HEADACHES

A stress or tension headache is the most common type of headache. These headaches can occur one or two times per month or more often, depending on your stress level. Reiki can reduce the pain of stress headaches and help you find the root cause of the stress.

❶ Drink eight ounces of pure water, then connect with Reiki in a dark, quiet room.

❷ Take a deep breath and exhale slowly. Then breathe normally and lie on your back. Close your eyes, place your hands together and cover the back of your head. Send Reiki to this area for 7 to 10 minutes or until the pain is gone.

❸ Stay in the quiet for an additional 10 minutes and just relax, breathing normally. (It is common to fall asleep at this point.)

❹ Repeat this sequence as necessary for pain. If this problem is frequent, journal what is causing the stress and how you feel about the situation. If the situation persists, meditate on how you can change or improve it.

FEAR

No one likes to be afraid or fearful. Reiki can help you better understand and control this emotional response.

1 Take a deep breath in through the nose and exhale slowly through the mouth like you are blowing out a candle. Repeat three times.

2 Breathe normally and check into Reiki. Lie back and move one hand to the inside of the opposite wrist and send energy for five to seven minutes.

3 Switch hands and repeat the procedure.

4 Stand up and Reiki the tailbone area for up to 10 minutes as you breathe normally and repeat the affirmation *I am safe*. Fearful feelings should have lessened by this time. End the session by drinking eight ounces of water and journaling your experience.

WORRY

Have you ever felt like you were stuck on a worry hamster wheel and couldn't break free? Everyone experiences this feeling from time to time. When we can't shut off our minds, worry takes over and robs us of living in the moment. Use this simple Reiki exercise to free yourself and return to the present moment.

1 Connect with Reiki and place your hands on your back. Begin with your hands lightly resting in the center of the back, one hand in front of the other. Follow this hand position all the way down the back, alternating which hand is in front, and spending about 10 minutes or as long as needed in each position.

2 If your mind wanders to catastrophic thinking during the session, stop and write down exactly what you are worried about. For every worry find a positive statement. For example, if you think *I am worried I will lose my job,* write a positive counter, such as *My job is secure.* Do this with everything that is worrying you, no matter how likely it is to happen or how much of an impact it will have on your life. Often when we worry about something large, like losing our source of income, we go down a rabbit hole, and many new worries pop up, like *How will I feed my fish if I lose my job?* Address all of these worries one by one.

❸ Place the power symbol on the back of the paper and find a safe place (such as a firepit, fireplace, or fireproof bowl) to burn the paper. Return to the Reiki session and start from the beginning. When we take the time to identify and write out what is bothering us, we see how unlikely it is to happen. We further release the fearful, worried thoughts by writing out the worries and burning the paper.

REIKI FOR EMOTIONAL SUPPORT

There are times when you may feel too sensitive or too emotional. Use this sequence with Reiki-infused tiger eye to help rebalance your energy and calm a stressed nervous system.

❶ Take a deep cleansing breath and check into Reiki.

❷ Begin by Reiking the back of the neck and behind the ears, beginning with the left side of the head and moving to the right. Spend at least 10 minutes in each position.

❸ Repeat the affirmation *I am strong and capable* as you move through the sequence. Spend as much time as needed in each position.

CONTINUED

④ Place a small piece of tiger eye outside in the moonlight (a full moon works best) for several nights and send Reiki to it. Once the stone has been infused with moonlight, carry it with you when you feel you need extra emotional support.

⑤ Continue to charge the stone in the moonlight and cleanse it as needed.

ANGER

Reiki can help you deal with and understand your anger. Often we are angry about a thing or an event, but it isn't really the root cause of the emotion.

① Begin by taking three deep breaths and slowly exhaling. Then continue breathing normally, but be aware of your breath.

② Check into Reiki and place your hands by the pubic bone. Angle your hands so they follow the groin. Send energy for 7 to 10 minutes.

③ Move one hand to the heart chakra and the other around the throat. Stay in this position for about 10 minutes or for as long as you are comfortable.

④ Finish this sequence off with one hand over the third eye chakra and the other hand on the back of the head. As your energy calms, note what images or memories come up.

⑤ Journal anything you thought of or any messages that came up and look for patterns.

⑥ Are you angry because someone found fault with your performance at work and told you what to do, but during the Reiki session you remembered that your parents used to do the same thing? If this is the case, send Reiki to the past event(s) using the long-distance symbol and write this entire experience out. Take your time to further examine what needs to be addressed and healed.

FOR FEELING OVERWHELMED

Are you feeling stressed out and overwhelmed? Reiki can help!

❶ Drink a glass of pure water and move to a quiet place where you will be alone and are not likely to be disturbed.

❷ Connect with Reiki and draw the power symbol once in the air above your body.

❸ Take three deep breaths and slowly release them. If possible, lie flat on your back and place both hands over your face or hover them one to two inches above your face. Cup your hands together and allow the Reiki to flow.

❹ After five to seven minutes, shift to a sitting position and Reiki the bottom of the feet. Send Reiki to the soles of the feet for 10 to 15 minutes or as needed.

❺ Sit in a meditative pose (one that is easy and comfortable). Place your hands at your sides or in your lap and sit quietly, allowing the energy to settle around you.

❻ End the session by clapping your hands and drinking at least another sip of water. Repeat as necessary throughout the day.

TO EASE A RACING MIND

If you are suffering from monkey mind, this sequence will help you settle down and calm your thoughts.

① If possible, find a place outside under a tree to perform this sequence. If the weather or your situation makes this impossible, sit quietly on the floor or on a yoga mat.

② Take a deep breath and release it slowly.

③ Check into Reiki. Place one hand on the brow; the other should cradle the back of the skull.

④ Allow the Reiki to flow as you quietly chant *Reiki, Reiki, Reiki* until your mind settles. You can chant out loud or in your mind.

⑤ Close your eyes, and in your mind's eye, see a red candle with a flame burning brightly. Concentrate on this flame as you chant. (This may take a few tries but do not become discouraged.)

⑥ Send energy for about 10 to 12 minutes or until the mind settles. Repeat as needed.

ACCEPTANCE

There are times when things don't work out as we had hoped, and we must learn to accept the situation. If you are having issues accepting something like a divorce, the loss of a job, or anything that has happened outside your control, this sequence might be beneficial for you.

❶ Begin in a room where you will not be disturbed for 20 to 30 minutes.

❷ Shut off all electronics and connect to Reiki.

❸ Close your eyes and take two deep cleansing breaths. Breathe in through the nose and slowly exhale through the mouth like you are blowing out a candle.

❹ Breathe normally and calmly as you open your eyes and stack your hands over the middle of the chest and Reiki the heart chakra area. Allow the energy to flow as you breathe normally for 10 minutes.

❺ While in this position, imagine your exhales are expelling all resistance, fear, or negative energy related to your situation. Every inhale is bringing in peace and understanding.

❻ Finish the session when you feel the energy has shifted.

❼ Journal your feelings associated with the session and enjoy a glass of water.

GUILT / SELF-LOATHING

If you are struggling with guilt and self-loathing, Reiki can help. We Reiki these chakras to ease guilt and issues related to self-loathing, self-destruction, and poor choices. Use the lessons from the past to make better decisions in the future, but let go of the guilt.

1. If possible, sit outside in nature. If this is not possible, sit either on the floor or in a chair with your bare feet touching the floor.
2. Take three deep cleansing breaths and release each slowly.
3. Sit in silence for a few seconds as you breathe normally.
4. Next, stand and Reiki the root chakra. Spend at least five to seven minutes on this energy center.
5. Move to the sacral chakra. Spend at least five to seven minutes or as much time as needed on this center.
6. Silently repeat the affirmation *I am healing as I release all anger, fear, excuses, and guilt completely.*

TO STORE POWER

The abdomen (tan tien in martial arts) is where many people believe we store spiritual energy. You may want to incorporate this energy session into your daily routine, after yoga, or before meditation or martial arts training.

1. Ground and center yourself.
2. Check into Reiki and place your hands on your stomach. You may notice a slight tingle or pull as the energy flows. Send Reiki for about 10 to 12 minutes per session. It is important to keep your mind focused and positive while you are doing this.
3. Repeat daily.

SPEAK YOUR TRUTH

If you are struggling with being authentic, feel judged because of your beliefs, or are fearful people will not accept you, then this sequence may change your life.

1 Face a mirror and ground yourself to the earth.

2 Check into Reiki.

3 Gently place your hands over the throat chakra and over the heart and send energy for five to seven minutes.

4 Look at your reflection in the mirror and smile.

5 Shift both hands to behind the head.

6 Move one hand to the neck and continue to send energy for as long as the chakra will take it.

7 Look at yourself in the mirror and repeat the affirmation *I easily speak my truth and I accept myself for who I am*. Repeat daily or as needed. (In the beginning you may not be comfortable looking at yourself in the mirror. That's okay, but try it anyway and stick with it. It will become easier the more you practice.)

RETURN TO JOY

If you are feeling like you lost your joy or like life is no longer an exciting adventure, try this sequence. Spend time taking care of yourself and doing something you love. We often lose our joy when we feel stressed out and overwhelmed. Begin journaling your thoughts every morning to understand what is causing this problem.

❶ If possible, sit quietly outside. If this is not practical for you, sit on a yoga mat inside a quiet room.

❷ Turn off all electronics and be fully aware and present as you connect with Reiki.

❸ Place your hands on the ankles, sending energy for five to seven minutes.

❹ Move to the bottom of the feet. Reiki each foot for at least 10 minutes. Repeat the affirmation *I step into a life of joy* throughout the session and upon waking every morning.

PEACEFUL NIGHT'S SLEEP

Did you know that one of the side effects of Reiki is sleeping like a baby? If you have trouble sleeping or if you wake up in the morning feeling exhausted, begin this sequence tonight.

❶ Just before bedtime, prepare for bed as normal and turn off the lights.

❷ Lie in your bed and check into Reiki.

❸ Place your hands on the crown of your head. Send Reiki for at least 10 minutes to this chakra as you repeat the affirmation *I enjoy a restful night's sleep and awake refreshed every morning.*

❹ Repeat nightly before bed.

CONTINUED

⑤ You may also want to place a piece of Reiki-infused lepidolite on your nightstand. If you are a crystal lover, you probably have a variety of stones throughout your living space. Make sure that you limit the number of stones by your bed or in your bedroom. Too many crystals and stones can interfere with your sleep cycle and keep you awake.

TO REMEMBER YOUR DREAMS

Reiki can empower your sleep and help you remember your dreams.

① Right before going to bed, write your intention to remember your dreams in a journal and place on your bedside table.

② Prepare for bed, turn off the lights, and lie down.

③ Get comfortable and connect with Reiki.

④ Place your hands on the sides of your head and send energy for 10 minutes.

⑤ Move to the third eye chakra and Reiki for five additional minutes.

⑥ Finish with your hands on the crown chakra for five to seven minutes and go to sleep.

⑦ As you feel yourself drifting off to sleep, repeat the intention that you will remember your dreams.

⑧ Keep your dream journal handy by the bed and make a habit of recording your dreams every morning before you get up. Soon you will be filling notebooks with your nightly adventures.

STIMULATE PHYSICAL HEALING

Our bodies are ready to heal, but occasionally they need a push, especially if we are out of alignment, overly stressed, or emotionally overwhelmed. Take the time to self-Reiki to give your body the energy it needs to heal.

① Take several deep breaths and slowly exhale.

② Breathe normally and sit comfortably on the floor with bare feet.

③ Reiki the sole of your left foot for about five minutes, then release your foot and move your hands to the right foot.

④ Reiki the bottom of this foot. Move from the toes down to the heel, giving special attention to the chakras in the pad and heel of the foot.

CONTINUED

⑤ After both feet have been given energy, make a fist with your dominant hand and lightly tap it against the sole of each foot, 29 times per foot. For maximum benefit, repeat this entire healing exercise daily.

EMPOWER YOURSELF

Are you feeling lost or without direction? Reiki can empower you and help you find your way.

❶ Begin by grounding with earth and placing a piece of selenite on your body. A beaded bracelet works best as it touches your skin and allows movement, but a raw piece on your lap or in your pocket will work.

❷ Check into Reiki. Take a deep, slow breath in and slowly exhale.

❸ Place your hands on your shoulder blades (do not cross your arms) for five to seven minutes. If you become stiff or uneasy in this position, move on to the next position.

4 Shift to the heart chakra for an additional 10 minutes.

5 Next, send Reiki to the bottom of each foot for five to seven minutes.

6 After the session, sit quietly and hold or wear the selenite. Think about what you would like to do in the next few years. Where would you like to go? What adventures would you like to have? Write everything in your journal.

ENHANCE YOUR CREATIVITY

Reiki can help you reconnect with your creativity in new and amazing ways! Repeat this sequence as needed to balance the third eye chakra and enhance your creativity.

1 Ground yourself and check into Reiki.

2 Take a deep breath and close your eyes. Imagine the power symbol is drawn on your palms.

3 Open your eyes and place your hands in the solar plexus position, under the breasts and over the lower ribs. Feel your palms activate as you send energy to this chakra. Stay here for 10 minutes.

4 Move your hands to the third eye chakra.

CONTINUED

5 Close your eyes and see golden light streaming down on you. As the light showers you, you should feel happy and empowered.

6 Repeat the affirmation *I am creative*.

GRATITUDE

As we begin to work with Reiki, the narrative of our life can shift and change. We may suddenly see our lives differently. For example, we may realize we were very lucky to have the parents, friends, or siblings we did growing up. Or we may suddenly see that our abilities, which we once considered curses, are actually gifts.

1 Check into Reiki and send energy to a rose quartz pendant, necklace, or stone.

2 Reiki the item with the intention that when wearing the piece, it will open your heart, and you will become more grateful.

3 Put the item on and repeat the affirmation *I am grateful for all I have* throughout the day.

STIMULATE
EMOTIONAL HEALING

Emotional healing is something that most people run away from. We are fearful of reliving past trauma and feeling all the turmoil associated with it. But in reality, we have already gone through and survived the situation. The only thing left is to heal it and finally be free from the past. We can begin this process with the assistance of Reiki.

1 Ground yourself into the earth and check into Reiki.

2 Place a piece of Reiki-infused rhodochrosite on your person. It can be worn or carried, but ideally the stone should touch your skin.

3 Repeat the affirmation *I am open to emotional healing for my highest good* daily.

4 Self-Reiki your heart chakra for five to seven minutes daily.

5 Journal any emotions or memories that come up to be healed. Do this without judgment as you allow yourself to feel the emotions that are associated with the situations.

6 Drink more water and rest more. Reassure yourself that you have nothing to fear now and release any tension or pain that comes up.

RELATIONSHIP ISSUES

Reiki can help us acknowledge, accept, and change our views on relationships. We ultimately cannot change anyone else, but we can change how we react to situations and become more aware of our own expectations. Are we expecting too much from someone else or are we settling for less than we deserve? With the help of Reiki, we can acknowledge our feelings and make the necessary changes to be in healthy, happy relationships.

❶ Ground yourself and connect to Reiki.

❷ Lightly place your hands in the middle of the back above the kidneys and send Reiki for as long as the chakra will take the energy.

❸ Switch your hands to the heart and throat, sending energy to these areas for at least 10 to 15 minutes.

❹ Imagine the relationship issues changing and healing. See yourself in the future happy with this relationship.

CLEAR ENERGY BLOCK IN LOWER BODY

If you are feeling sluggish or grumpy, or you're tired in the morning even after a full night's sleep and feel fearful for no logical reason, you could have a lower-body energy block.

❶ Drink eight to ten ounces of pure water. After you finish the water, ground yourself to the earth.

❷ Check into Reiki.

❸ Sit down in a comfortable position either on the floor or in a chair. Place one hand above the kneecap and the other under the knee and send Reiki.

❹ Repeat on other leg, spending at least 15 minutes on each knee.

5 Finish the session off with a nap or warm bath, if possible. Taking a warm bath or shower will further release any energy blocks after this session. If a nap or bath is not possible, sit quietly and allow your energy to rebalance before you do anything strenuous or taxing.

6 Repeat daily as needed.

GROUNDING BEFORE SPIRIT WORK

It is always wise to be 100 percent present, focused, and grounded before participating in any type of spiritual work. This is important for a number of reasons, including your safety. Reiki can assist you in staying centered, empowered, and calm during these sessions and help you recover afterward.

1 To ease tension and build focus before any type of spirit work, check into Reiki and ground yourself in whatever manner makes the most sense to you.

2 Next, place one hand over the sole of your bare foot. Place the other hand over the top of the foot and Reiki for about 10 minutes.

3 Switch to the other foot and repeat the process. If you find you are losing your focus, repeat as needed.

TO SOOTHE EMPATHS OR EMPATHY OVERLOAD

In this day and age, it is very easy to become overwhelmed by all the emotional news stories we are exposed to. When you feel especially emotional or if you know you are an empath, you may want to include this sequence in your weekly self-care routine.

1. Find a quiet and private place, free from electronics, where you will not be disturbed.

2. Ground yourself fully and check into Reiki.

3. Take several deep cleansing breaths and allow your shoulders to droop as you breathe normally.

4. Place a piece of Reiki-infused rose quartz in your pocket, bra, or clothing. You may use a piece of jewelry or a raw stone for this exercise.

5. Gently Reiki the throat chakra for at least five to seven minutes.

6. Move your hands to the collarbone and Reiki for at least five to seven minutes.

7. Finish by sending energy to the heart. Stay in this position for at least 10 minutes or for as long as the area pulls energy.

8. Repeat as needed and include more quiet time in your routine. Spend some time unplugged from social media and people to recharge.

FOR FOCUS AND CONCENTRATION

Reiki can help you calm your mind and become much more focused. If you know you have a test or something that needs your full concentration coming up, begin this sequence one week to one day before the event.

1. Find a quiet place and ground yourself to the earth.
2. Check into Reiki and begin with your hands at the side of the head, slightly cupping your ears. Stay in this position as long as it's comfortable.
3. Move your hands to the shoulder/collarbone area and continue to send energy.
4. Clear your mind and allow the Reiki to flow with no direction or intended outcome. Repeat the affirmation *I have great focus and concentration*.
5. Drink at least eight ounces of cold water and begin your task.
6. Repeat as needed.

STRENGTHEN INTUITION

Just being attuned to Reiki will strengthen your intuition, but if you want to jump-start it even more, try this simple exercise. Visit a crystal shop (in person is best, but online will work, too). Look for high vibrational stones like celestite, moldavite, iolite, or ametrine for this sequence. Pick the stone that feels right to you and follow these steps.

1. Once you have your stone, place it in a bowl and cover it fully with uncooked rice. Allow it to stay in the rice one full week.
2. After one week, uncover the stone and throw the rice away. (Do NOT eat the rice or feed it to pets.)
3. Send Reiki to the stone or place it outside in the moonlight to charge.
4. Once the stone is charged, wear it daily and sleep with it under your pillow.

CONTINUED

⑤ Working with higher vibrational, Reiki-infused stones can open up many new psychic gifts. But a word of warning—moldavite can cause headaches and anxiety until you become used to the energy, so if you are new to working with crystals, begin with one of the other stones.

ENHANCE YOUR CONNECTION WITH YOUR GUIDES

Everyone has at least one guide. Some guides are with us our entire lives, and others are only here to help us through certain experiences. By connecting with Reiki and aligning your chakras, you will soon be able to interact with the world in a whole new way.

❶ Ground and center yourself.
❷ Take a few deep breaths and release any judgments or conceptions about what is supposed to happen when you connect with guides.
❸ After connecting with Reiki, place your hands on your face, covering your eyes. Do not put any pressure on your face. Allow the Reiki to flow and keep your mind neutral.
❹ After 10 minutes, move your hands to the sides of your face, covering your ears. Repeat the affirmation *I am open to divine guidance*.

⑤ Move to Reiki the top of the head.

⑥ You may not hear or see anything during the Reiki session. (But you might!) Your guide will probably connect with you via music, repeating messages or numbers, or dreams.

⑦ Journal everything that happens after the session.

REIKI FOR POSITIVE THOUGHTS

If you feel overwhelmed by negative thoughts, try this sequence.

❶ Connect to Reiki and send energy to the root chakra for as long as it will take the energy.

❷ Next, place your hand behind you and Reiki the hara chakra on your back, repeating the process of offering energy for as long as the chakra takes the energy.

❸ Sit down comfortably and place a piece of Reiki-infused turquoise in your right hand. Place that hand, gripping the stone, over your heart.

CONTINUED

④ Close your eyes and visualize yourself being happy. See yourself laughing, smiling, and having fun. Note what you are doing, where you are, what you are you wearing, and who is with you.

⑤ Sit with this energy for up to 20 minutes and then journal everything you saw.

⑥ Repeat daily as need.

AUTOMATIC WRITING

Automatic writing is a form of channeling higher realms of energy and consciousness. If you want to connect with Spirit for guidance, then this is an easy exercise to try.

① Ground yourself and spend about five minutes sending energy to each hand.

② Next, Reiki your pencil and paper.

③ Set your intention. Say something like, *I will become a clear writing channel for Spirit, and I allow myself the space to write without ego.*

④ Begin your session with an open mind, free from preconceived ideas of what you think should happen.

⑤ Set a timer for 10 minutes and write freely without editing or reading your work.

⑥ When the timer goes off, go back and read what you have written. It may take a bit of practice, but this is a great way to connect with Spirit.

CONNECT WITH YOUR INNER CHILD

The child you once were is still inside you, no matter what age you are today. Chances are that they are still wanting to play, explore, and learn. But it is also likely that unhealed trauma from childhood is weighing heavily on your inner child. We can begin to heal this pain and free ourselves by working with Reiki.

① Connect to Reiki and place your hands in the middle of your stomach, around the belly button.

② After 10 minutes, move to the heart chakra.

③ Repeat the affirmation *My inner child is safe and loved* during the session.

④ Be open to whatever images or emotions come up and do not judge yourself.

⑤ Journal your experience and repeat this exercise weekly.

CONNECT WITH YOUR ANCESTORS

When we are feeling stuck and in need of clarity, our ancestors are always there to support us.

❶ Ground and connect to Reiki.

❷ Sit down and begin with the palms on the instep of the foot as it meets the ball of the foot. Reiki the feet for about nine minutes.

❸ Close your eyes as you move through the sequence and repeat the affirmation *I seek to connect with my ancestors*.

❹ Move your hands to the crease at the top of the thighs.

❺ After 10 minutes, move to the heart chakra and Reiki for five to seven minutes.

❻ Move to the crown chakra and Reiki for five to seven minutes.

❼ Do not judge any images or information that enters your mind.

❽ Journal your results and limit this practice to once per week. Note any dreams, repeating patterns, or surprises you have in the days following this exercise.

KUNDALINI BREATHING AND REIKI

Breath work and Reiki work very well together.

1 Ground yourself and Reiki each foot from a sitting or lying position for about seven minutes.

2 Lie on your back and send Reiki to your body by placing one hand on your heart chakra and the other below your rib cage.

3 Breathe in slowly through your nose and feel your stomach expand under your hand. The hand sending Reiki to your heart should be as still as possible. Watch your breathing and fill the lungs fully on each inhale.

4 Stay in this position, breathing mindfully for 5 to 10 minutes. This sequence should activate your Kundalini and should be practiced with care. Don't overdo this practice.

CONNECTING TO HIGHER CONSCIOUSNESS

Reiki can assist us in connecting to a state of higher consciousness.

1 Ground yourself and connect to Reiki.

2 Send energy to your third eye chakra for 7 to 10 minutes.

3 Move your hands to the crown chakra and Reiki for 10 minutes.

4 Next, sit in meditation and place a piece of Reiki-infused amethyst in each hand.

5 Clear your mind and allow the experience to unfold.

6 Sit for at least 30 minutes.

7 Note any messages, visions, or beings you see in your journal. Connecting to higher consciousness can be taxing on the physical body. Drink plenty of water and rest after each session.

8 Repeat no more than once per week.

CHANTING TO STRENGTHEN YOUR CONNECTION TO REIKI

Chanting the names of the Reiki symbols in meditation is one of the easiest ways to work with them.

1 Check into Reiki and sit in quiet meditation for a few moments with your hands in front of you as if in prayer.

2 When you are ready, with eyes closed, chant softly. Begin by chanting only the power symbol for a few days before adding the long-distance symbol.

3 If you wish to begin an emotional healing session, you may say the name of the mental/emotional symbol, but be warned, it could bring up past trauma and unlock an avalanche of emotions.

REIKI AND YOGA

Reiki works in tandem with yoga for deep healing. There are many ways to connect Reiki to your yoga practice.

1 Connect to Reiki and give each knee a quick Reiki treatment.

2 Move to Reiki the feet and then begin yoga poses.

3 You can also Reiki yourself and move into the half lotus position on a yoga mat. In this position, your legs are crossed with one foot resting on the opposite thigh. The other foot folds underneath the top leg and rests below the knee or thigh.

4 Sit in quiet meditation and allow the Reiki to flow through the body.

REIKI FOR LUCID DREAMING

Entering the lucid or conscious dreaming state takes practice, but Reiki, combined with crystals, can help you relax into the correct mindset.

1 Place several pieces of Reiki-infused amethyst, fluorite, and quartz on your nightstand before bed. These should be small, tumbled stones, not large pieces.

2 Give yourself a mini-Reiki session 30 minutes before bed.

3 Lie comfortably in your bed and send Reiki to both feet for three to five minutes.

4 Reiki the ankles for an additional three minutes.

5 Place your hands on your tailbone and Reiki the root chakra for five to seven minutes.

6 Close your eyes and move your hands to the throat chakra. Send energy for five minutes.

7 Move your hands to the third eye position and send energy for five minutes or as needed.

8 Move your hands to the crown chakra and send energy as you set the intention that you will wake up in your dreams and know that you are dreaming.

9 Keep a dream journal handy to record your dreams. With continued practice, you will soon notice amazing results.

ACCESS HIDDEN MEMORIES

It is common to have hidden or repressed memories. They could be from childhood or past lives. Accessing these hidden memories may give you answers or explanations, but it is important to remember that we live in the present and not become connected to the past.

① Check into Reiki and close your eyes.

② Place one hand on the back of the head at the vagus nerve area, just above where the neck joins the head. Place your other hand across the forehead. Send Reiki for 7 to 10 minutes.

③ Allow your mind to calm. While breathing normally, see in your mind's eye the long-distance symbol floating before you. Imagine it settling on your third eye chakra.

④ Move your hands to the back of the head. With your little fingers touching beneath your head, cup the area of your head where the occipital lobe is located. Send Reiki for another 7 to 10 minutes. The long-distance symbol combined with the hand sequence may trigger memories from this life or others. Journal everything, stay hydrated, and rest afterward.

⑤ Don't rush to repeat this sequence; it is important to give your mind and body time to process these memories before the next session.

REIKI TO CLEAR OUT STALE, STUCK, AND STAGNANT ENERGY

If you feel stuck or "off" and have no idea how you ended up feeling like this, it could be because you are carrying around stagnant energy. We literally drag this energy around behind us like a heavy sack filled with cement. It weights us down and saps our energy, along with our joy. Use Reiki to release this energy and feel good again!

1 Take a deep breath and settle down.

2 Connect to Reiki and envision a silver liquid energy moving down the spine as you place one hand on the back of the neck and the other on the base of the spine. Allow the energy to flow the length of the spine, cleaning and healing as it goes. Allow it to remove old thought forms, outdated ideas, and habits that are stuck. Stay quietly in this position, envisioning the energy moving down your spine for at least five minutes or for as long as needed.

3 Stay calm and allow this energy to work and repeat the affirmation *I release all stuck, stale, and stagnant energy that no longer serves my highest good.*

4 Finish the session off with a glass of water and, if possible, a nap. If you are not able to sleep, sit quietly for 10 minutes more as the energy continues to clear out old debris. You might also want to soak in a warm bath or take a shower after this session.

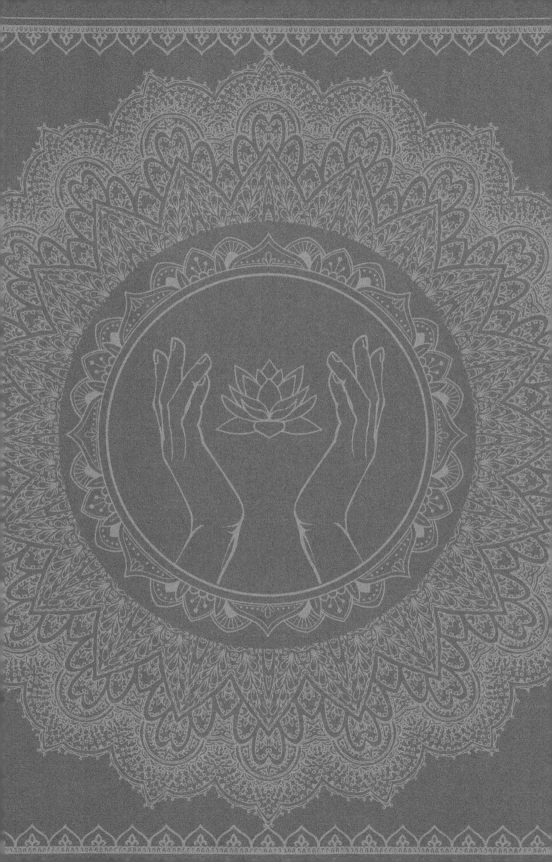

Resources

http://www.serenityreikiclinic.com
This is the website for my Reiki clinic, where you can learn about everyday uses for Reiki and more.

http://www.sarahparkerthomas.com
This is the website for my spiritual coaching. You can learn more here about combining Reiki with other healing modalities.

https://iarp.org
This website is a great source of reference material for anyone wanting to know more about Reiki.

http://www.reiki.nu/index.html
This website lists easy hand positions for common alignments.

https://jpninfo.com/37451
Visit this website to learn more about kotodama and the power of words.

https://www.rd.com/culture/smiley-face-invented/
Visit this site to learn more about symbols in culture, especially the smiley face.

References

Melody. *Love Is in the Earth: A Kaleidoscope of Crystals; The Updated Reference Book Describing the Metaphysical Properties of the Mineral Kingdom*. Portland, ME: Earth Love Publishing House, 2003.

Index

A

Acceptance, 136
Anxiety, 126
Ascension symptoms, 115–116
Astral projection, 40
Attunement, 3, 10–11, 53
Auras, 41, 42, 98
Authenticity, 138

B

Balance, 34, 35
Black obsidian, 65
Breath work, 69–70, 155.
    See also Pranayamas

C

Chakra meditations, 68–69
Chakras, 16, 18–19, 35, 106.
    See also specific
Chanting, 157
Chi (energy), 9
Children, 23, 27
Clairaudience, 38
Clairsentience, 38
Clairvoyance, 38, 47–49
Classes, 58. See also Teachers
Complementary practices, 63–71
Concentration, 149
Consent, 22–23
Creativity, 143–144
Crown chakra, 18, 105–106
Crystals, 64–65

D

Distance healing, 21–22
Dreams, 40, 140–141. See also
    Lucid dreaming

E

Emotional/spiritual healing
    sequences, 125
acceptance, 136
access hidden memories, 159
anger, 132–133
automatic writing, 152–153
chanting to strengthen your
    connection to Reiki, 157
clear energy block in lower
    body, 146–147
connecting to higher
    consciousness, 156
connect with your ancestors, 154
connect with your inner child, 153
ease a racing mind, 135
empower yourself, 142–143
enhance your connection with your
    guides, 150–151
enhance your creativity, 143–144
fear, 129
for feeling overwhelmed, 134
for focus and concentration, 149
gratitude, 144
grief, 127
grounding before spirit work, 147
guilt/self-loathing, 137
Kundalini breathing and Reiki, 155
peaceful night's sleep, 139–140
Reiki and yoga, 157
Reiki for emotional support, 131–132
Reiki for lucid dreaming, 158
Reiki for positive thoughts, 151–152
Reiki to clear out stale, stuck, and
    stagnant energy, 160
relationship issues, 146
release anxiety, 126
remember your dreams, 140–141

return to joy, 139
for shielding, 126
soothe empaths or empathy
    overload, 148
speak your truth, 138
stimulate emotional healing, 145
stimulate physical healing, 141–142
store power, 137
strengthen intuition, 149–150
stress headaches, 128
worry, 130–131
Empaths, 33, 36, 37, 148
Empowerment, 142–143
Energy, 7, 9, 56. *See also* Chakras
Energy healing. *See* Healing
Essential oils, 65–66
Ethics, 56–57

F

Fear, 129
Feet chakras, 19, 96
Flow, 31
Fluorite, 65
Focus, 149

G

Gassho, 4, 69
Gratitude, 144
Grief, 127
Guides, 42–43, 150–151
Guilt, 137

H

Hand chakras, 19
Hand positions, 21–22. *See also*
    Emotional/spiritual healing
    sequences; Sequences
ankles, for energy blockages, 95
ankles, for self-healing, 80
back of head, for self-healing, 76
crown, 85
crown, for self-healing, 76
ears, for self-healing, 77

elbows, 93
eyes, for self-healing, 77
face, 86
face, for self-healing, 77
for general well-being, 97
head, 84
heart, 89
heart, for self-healing, 78
knees, 94
knees, for self-healing, 80
lower stomach, 91
mid-back, for self-healing, 79
navel, for self-healing, 79
Reiki the hands, 92
rib cage, for self-healing, 78
smooth the client's aura, 98
solar plexus, for self-healing, 79
soles of the feet, for self-healing, 80
stomach, 90
temples, for self-healing, 76
throat, 88
throat, for self-healing, 78
top of the shoulder, 87
unblock a foot chakra, 96
Hara chakra, 18
Hayashi, Chujiro, 5
Hayashi Reiki Kenkyukai, 5
Healing. *See also* Emotional/spiritual
        healing sequences; Hand
        positions; Self-healing;
        Sequences
    about, 15–16
    benefits of, 44
    distance, 21–22
    group, 27
    hands-on, 21
    modalities, 6–7, 9, 63
    others, 26–27, 83, 99
    sessions, 28–29
    spiritual, 45
    as a spiritual practice, 34–35
    yourself, 26
Heart chakra, 17, 103

I

Illusions, 39
Inclusivity, 64
Intuitive abilities, 33, 36–37, 50–57,
    111–112, 149–150

J

Journaling, 48
Joy, 139

K

Ki (energy), 9
Kundalini yoga, 67–68

L

Lavender essential oil, 66
Lemon essential oil, 66
Letting go, 49
Long-distance symbol (Ho Sha Ze
    Sho Nen), 25
Lucid dreaming, 40, 158

M

Malachite, 65
Masters, 13
Master symbol (Dai Ko Myo), 25
Medical intuition, 41
Meditation, 53, 56, 68–69
Mediumship, 39–40
Memories, repressed, 159
Mental/emotional symbol
    (Sei He Ki), 24
Monkey mind, 135

N

Negative thoughts, 151–152

O

Okuden (Level 2), 12
Openness, 48
Out-of-body experiences, 40
Overwhelm, 134

P

Pets, 23, 27
Post-traumatic stress disorder, 118
Power symbol (Cho Ku Rei), 24
Practice environment, 51
Prana (energy), 9
Pranayamas, 68
Precepts, 4
Psychic abilities, 36, 38
Psychic fatigue, 60

Q

Qi (energy), 9
Quieting the mind, 49

R

Reiki
    basics, 6–7
    benefits of, 34
    history of, 3–5
    levels of, 11–13
    modern approaches to, 5–6
    precepts, 4
    prerequisite to performing, 10
    recipients of, 23
    spiritual, 9–10
Reiki boxes, 22
Reiki grids, 22
Relationship issues, 146
Root chakra, 16, 102
Rose quartz, 64

S

Sacral chakra, 17, 102
Sandalwood essential oil, 66
Self-care, 55, 60–61
Self-healing, 26, 44, 54–55, 75.
    See also Emotional/spiritual
        healing sequences; Sequences
    ankles hand position, 80
    back of head hand position, 76
    crown hand position, 76

ears hand position, 77
eyes hand position, 77
face hand position, 77
heart hand position, 78
knees hand position, 80
mid-back hand position, 79
navel hand position, 79
rib cage hand position, 78
solar plexus hand position, 79
soles of the feet hand position, 80
temples hand position, 76
throat hand position, 78
Self-loathing, 137
Seppuku (ritual suicide), 5
Sequences. See also Emotional/
    spiritual healing sequences
to access past-life memories, 117
for ascension symptoms, 115
for balancing personal energy, 114
for building your intuitive
    muscles—feeling, 112
for building your intuitive
    muscles—seeing, 111
chakra clearing energy
    pathways, 106
before channeling, 120
connect to angelic beings, 113
before craft/spell work, 119
crown chakra support, 105–106
heart chakra support, 103
for manifesting, 122–123
for manifesting a positive
    outcome, 109
for mental/emotional ascension
    symptoms, 116
to move forward, 110
post-traumatic stress disorder, 118
for restoring the body after a
    spiritual experience, 108–109
root chakra support, 102
sacral chakra support, 102
for self-awareness, 121
solar plexus chakra support, 103
for spiritual awakening, 107

before a tarot reading, 118
third eye chakra support, 104–105
throat chakra support, 104
Sessions, 28–29
Shinpiden (Levels 3 and 4), 13
Shoden (Level 1), 11–12
Signs, 49
Sleep, 139–140
Smoky quartz, 65
Solar plexus chakra, 17, 103
Spiritual awakenings, 52–53
Spiritual experiences, 8, 29, 31–36, 49.
    See also Sequences
Spiritual guides, 42–43, 150–151
Spiritual healing. See Emotional/
    spiritual healing sequences
Stress, 128
Surrogates, 22
Symbols, 24–25
Synchronicity, 36

T
Takata, Hawayo, 5
Takata, Mrs., 5, 24
Teachers, 13, 58–60, 71
Third eye chakra, 18, 47–49, 104–105
Throat chakra, 17, 104

U
Usui, Mikao, 3–4, 5, 24

V
Visions, 38–39

W
Wicca, 70–71
Witchcraft, 70–71
Worry, 130–131

Y
Yin yoga, 67
Yoga, 66–68, 157

Acknowledgments

This book would not have been possible without the support and encouragement of my son, Dylan Mercer, who has always believed in me and the miracle of Reiki.

I'm forever indebted to Lady Roxanna, Amanda Hart, Darryl Kempster, Cari Hyde, Angela Gonzales, Sarah Davidson, Debbie Hearn, Frank Hipchen, and Rochelle Cooney for their encouragement and ongoing support on this journey.

Words cannot express my gratitude to editor Clara Song Lee for her professional advice and assistance with this book. Also, thanks to everyone on the publishing team. You rock!

Any and all errors or omissions are mine. There is always so much more that could be said about this wondrous energy.

Reiki Blessings,

Sarah

About the Author

Sarah Parker Thomas was born in Gonzales, Texas, and has lived and studied in the UK and Europe. As an empath, she has had a lifelong interest in healing and helping others. Sarah is a Reiki master sensei, a Bliss Soul 2 Soul spiritual coach, a master of manifesting, a lucid dreaming healer, and a renowned energy healer. She is also an author, a teacher, and the owner of Serenity Reiki Clinic.

Many people count Sarah as a shaman for her lifelong study of the healing arts, both with indigo people and abroad. She continues to build on her knowledge and hands-on skills with multiple energy modalities and her devotion to helping others lead healthy, stress-free lives. She has had a lifelong interest in healing; has studied nutrition, earth energies, traditional Chinese medicine, and yoga; and has been active in her community as an elected official, a board member for children's advocacy, and a business owner. Sarah actively supports the arts and animal rights, and volunteers her time around the world.

CPSIA information can be obtained
at www.ICGtesting.com
Printed in the USA
JSHW011119220520
5770JS00001BA/2